DEPROGRAMMING
AND
REPROGRAMMING
OF THE MIND

TAKE THE VEGAN OATH

HI MY NAME IS _____
AND I WAS A FLESH EATER.

WELCOME TO THE WONDERFUL
JOURNEY OF A VEGAN LIFESTYLE

ISBN: 979-8-218-24134-6 - Paperback

Disclaimer

You will see this throughout this guide as a reminder. The information contained in this book is not intended to be a substitute for professional medical advice, diagnosis, or treatment. The author of this book is not a licensed doctor, practitioner, or nutritionist and the content provided is for informational purposes only. It is recommended that readers consult with a licensed healthcare professional before making any significant changes to their diet or lifestyle, especially if they have any underlying health conditions. The author cannot be held responsible for any outcomes resulting from the use of the information provided in this book. The reader assumes full responsibility for any actions taken based on the information presented.

LETTER FROM THE AUTHOR

I think it's fantastic that you've made the decision to go vegan. It's a courageous and compassionate choice that can have a positive impact not only on your own health, but also on the environment and animal welfare. I know it can be difficult to make a change like this, especially if it goes against the norm in your social circle or community.

I remember my own journey towards veganism wasn't a walk in the park. It took me a good 6 years to fully embrace this lifestyle and that too, not without skepticism and questioning looks from quite a few. One of the biggest challenges was finding helpful resources. I did not know where to begin. This is why my goal with this guide is to be the friend who can not only introduce you to this lifestyle but also walk you through the why's, how's, and what's of veganism.

But by choosing to follow your heart and your values, you're making a difference in the world and setting an example for others to follow. Keep up the great work and never forget why you started on this path. Remember that every time you choose plant-based options, you're making a powerful statement about what you believe in and how you want to live your life. You're doing amazing things for yourself and for your family, and I'm proud of you!

~Eva

CONTENTS

INTRODUCTION

Welcome to your Complete Guide to Everything You Need to Know to Go Vegan. This comprehensive book is designed to help you navigate the world of veganism with ease, covering all aspects of this increasingly popular way of life. Whether you're curious about the benefits of veganism or ready to take the plunge and make the switch, this guide is for you!

From understanding the definition of veganism and the ethical and environmental reasons why people choose this lifestyle, to practical tips on vegan food, diet, and nutrition, this guide has got you covered. I will also provide delicious vegan recipes to help you get started on your plant-based journey.

I understand that making the transition to a vegan lifestyle can be challenging, which is why I address common obstacles that many people face when making this change. This guide also provides answers to frequently asked questions about veganism to help you feel confident in your decision.

Additionally, I share personal insights into how I transitioned to a vegan lifestyle, offering inspiration and motivation to help you on your own journey. I believe that living a vegan lifestyle is not only great for your health, but also for the planet and the animals we share it with.

Thank you for choosing my vegan transition guide as your go-to resource for all things plant-based. I am so excited to support you on your journey towards a healthier, more sustainable lifestyle! Without further ado, let's dive in!

CHAPTER 1:
PREPARING YOUR MIND: MAKING THE TRANSITION

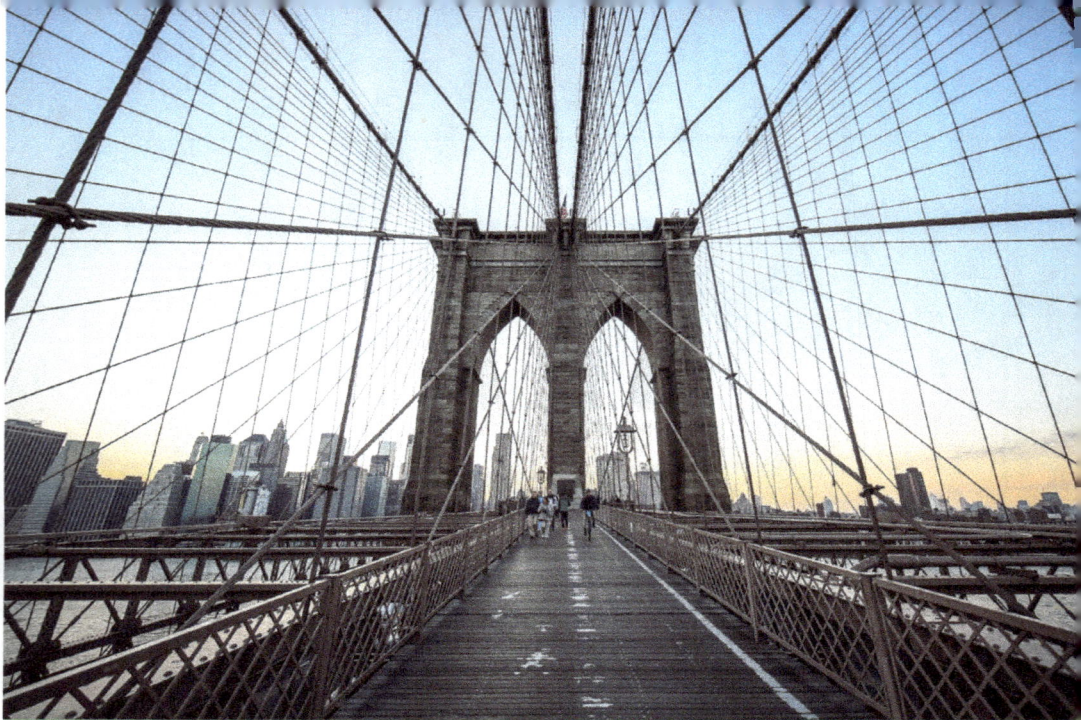

Making the transition to a vegan diet can be challenging, but with a little bit of planning and preparation, it can be made much easier. I wish someone had given me the following tips when I was getting started. They can save hours of wasted time and effort (and last-minute runs to the grocery store.)

1. **Plan your meals**

   One of the best ways to ensure that you stick to a vegan diet is to plan your meals in advance. This will help you avoid the temptation to reach for non-vegan options when you're hungry and in a rush. Start by making a list of vegan recipes that you want to try and then plan out your meals for the week.

2. **Stock up on staples**

   Staples are essential, basic foods that are commonly consumed in a particular diet or cuisine. In other words, these are the must-haves in your pantry. In a vegan diet, these may include plant-based foods such as beans, lentils, rice, quinoa, potatoes, sweet potatoes, bananas, apples, carrots, onions, and leafy greens. Basically, they can serve as the foundation of many meals and can be easily incorporated into a variety of recipes. Stock up on these items so that you have the basics covered.

3. **Explore new ingredients**

One of the best things about going vegan is that it'll force you to step out of your comfort zone, explore new ingredients and try new recipes. Experiment with different fruits, vegetables, grains, and legumes to keep your meals interesting and satisfying.

Exploring new ingredients can be a fun and exciting way to add variety and nutrition to your vegan diet. I was introduced to a whole world of culinary possibilities when starting out as a vegan. There are many plant-based foods out there that you may not have tried before, such as jackfruit, tempeh, nutritional yeast, and tofu. You can also experiment with different grains, like quinoa or farro, or different types of exotic fruits and veggies like dragon fruit or Bok choy.

Trying new ingredients can help you discover new flavors and textures and can also provide you with a wider range of nutrients to support your overall health and well-being. So, don't be afraid to get creative in the kitchen and try something new!

4. **Shop at farmer's markets**

This one is a multi-benefit tip. Farmer's markets are a great place to find fresh fruits and vegetables that are in season. Not only are they often more affordable than supermarket produce, but you'll also be supporting local farmers.

Farmers markets often have a wider variety of fruits and vegetables than you might find at a traditional grocery store, and they can also be a great place to find rare or unique ingredients. When you shop at a farmers' market, you're also reducing your carbon footprint by buying locally grown produce that doesn't have to travel long distances.

A few things I learnt from my frequent visits to many different farmers' markets: Before you go, do a little research on what's in season so you know what to look for. Bring reusable bags or containers with you, as many farmers markets don't provide plastic bags, and be prepared to pay with cash or card depending on the vendor's preference. Don't be afraid to ask questions or try samples and remember to be respectful of the farmers and their products. Shopping at a farmers' market can be a fun and educational experience, and it's a great way to connect with your community and support sustainable agriculture.

5. **Read labels carefully**

When shopping for packaged foods, be sure to read the labels carefully to ensure that they are vegan! For beginners, this can be a tricky one to navigate. Look for products that are labeled "vegan" or "plant-based" and check the ingredient list to ensure that there are no animal products or byproducts. If you're shopping for vegan products at a farmers' market, it's important to read labels carefully to make sure that what you're buying fits your dietary preferences. Many vendors will have signs or labels indicating which products are vegan, but it's always a good idea to double check.

Look for ingredients like animal byproducts (such as milk, eggs, or honey), as well as any products that may have been processed with animal-derived ingredients. Some fruits and vegetables may also be sprayed with non-vegan pesticides, so it's important to ask vendors about their growing practices if you have any concerns.

If you're not sure whether a product is vegan-friendly, don't hesitate to ask the vendor for more information. They may be able to provide you with a complete list of ingredients or recommend similar products that are vegan. By taking the time to read labels and ask questions, you can ensure that you're making informed choices and supporting sustainable agriculture practices.

I understand and know that making the transition to a vegan diet can seem slight intimidating in the start but it's all about taking baby steps. With some planning and preparation, it's perfectly doable. These tips will help you be on your way to a healthy and satisfying vegan lifestyle in no time!

CHAPTER 2:
WHAT IS VEGANISM, VEGETARIANISM AND PESCATARIANISM?

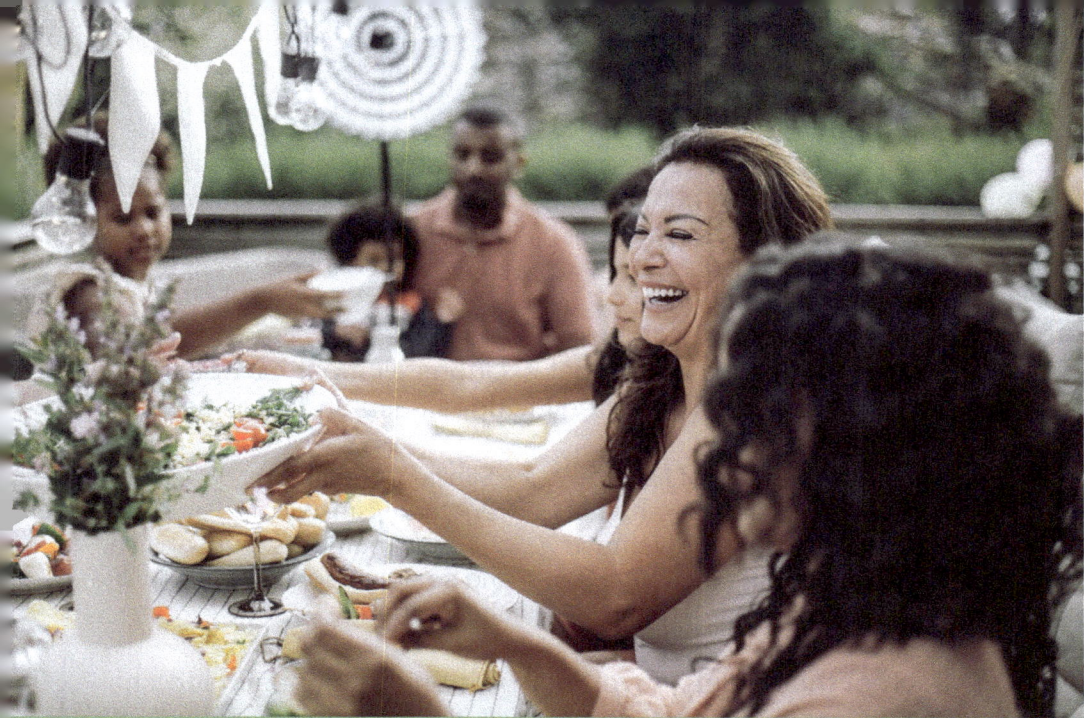

Veganism, **Vegetarianism** and **Pescatarianism** are all diets that involve the exclusion of certain types of animal products.

Veganism is a lifestyle that excludes all animal products, including meat, dairy, eggs, honey and even some clothing and personal care items made with animal products or tested on animals.

- Lowers risk of heart disease, high blood pressure, and type 2 diabetes

- Improved digestion and gut health

- Possible weight loss

- Lower risk of certain types of cancer

Vegetarianism excludes meat but may still include dairy and eggs. Some vegetarians also choose to exclude other animal products such as honey.

- Similar benefits to veganism, but with the added potential benefits of dairy and eggs (such as improved bone health from calcium in dairy products)

- Easier to maintain adequate protein intake for those who are not comfortable with a fully vegan diet

Pescatarianism is a diet that excludes all meat except for fish and seafood. This diet often includes dairy and eggs as well.

- Potential benefits of fish and seafood, such as omega-3 fatty acids which can improve heart health and brain function

- Similar benefits to vegetarianism, with the addition of certain nutrients found in fish and seafood (such as vitamin D and iodine).

Each of these diets have their own unique benefits and challenges, and the best choice will depend on an individual's beliefs, lifestyle and nutritional needs. It's always important to consult with a healthcare professional before making any major changes to your diet.

I can tell you from personal experience, seeking professional advice is important! Your healthcare provider can help you determine what types of foods and nutrients you need to support your overall health and well-being. They may also be able to provide you with resources and guidance on how to make healthy dietary changes that meet your individual needs.

CHAPTER 3:
ADDRESSING COMMON CONCERNS AND MISCONCEPTIONS ABOUT VEGANISM

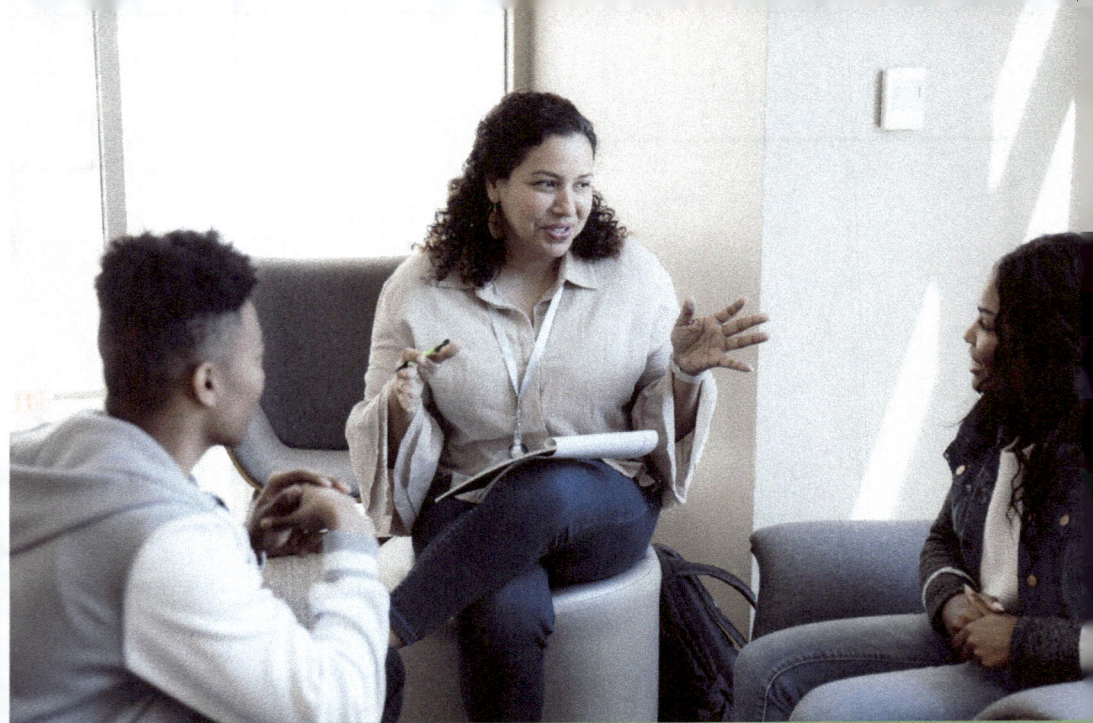

What I have usually seen from experience is that people are reluctant about veganism or stay away from even considering it as an alternative way of life because of the various myths and misconceptions attached to the concept. This is like missing out on a beautiful journey just because of a few false rumors about the destination.

Going vegan can be challenging for some people, as it may require significant changes in their dietary habits and lifestyle. However, with the right approach and mindset, it is achievable and can even be enjoyable. Don't get me wrong, it may take some time to learn about new ingredients and cooking methods, but there are plenty of resources available to help you on your journey.

In fact, what was more difficult for me was finding vegan options when dining out or attending social events. This requires some planning ahead and being comfortable asking for modifications or substitutions when ordering. In addition, there may be some cravings or social pressure to go back to old eating habits, but staying committed to your values and health goals can help overcome these challenges.

Overall, going vegan can be a positive and rewarding experience, both for your health and for the environment. It may take some effort and patience, but the benefits are worth it.

Now coming over to some misconceptions and myths. One common misconception is that veganism is a restrictive and unpalatable diet. However, with proper planning and preparation, vegans can enjoy a diverse and delicious array of plant-based foods. Another misconception is that veganism is not nutritionally complete, but a well-planned vegan diet can easily meet all the recommended dietary requirements.

I have realized that the best way to educate others about their dietary choices, is to engage in respectful and informative conversations, share resources such as books or documentaries, and lead by example through one's own healthy and compassionate lifestyle.

It is important for vegans to approach these conversations with an open mind and willingness to listen to others' perspectives, while also advocating for their own beliefs and values. Ultimately, education and awareness are key in helping to dispel misconceptions and promote understanding and acceptance of the vegan lifestyle.

Adam the Pro Athlete:

Meet Adam, a professional athlete who has been at the top of his game for years. He's won countless awards and accolades in football, but as he's gotten older, he's become increasingly concerned about his health. He's heard about the benefits of a vegan diet, but he's always been skeptical - he's worried that giving up meat and dairy will hurt his recovery time, make it harder to maintain his muscle mass, and ultimately hurt his performance on the field.

But after doing some research and talking to some other athletes who have successfully made the switch to a plant-based diet, Adam starts to reconsider. He realizes that with the right planning and preparation, he can still get all the nutrients and protein he needs to stay strong and healthy.

Adam starts by consulting with a registered dietitian who specializes in vegan nutrition. Together, they come up with a meal plan that is tailored to his specific needs - high in protein, but also rich in complex carbohydrates, healthy fats, and plenty of fruits and vegetables. Adam starts experimenting with new recipes and ingredients, like tofu, tempeh, and lentils, and finds that he enjoys the variety and flavors of his new diet.

In order to ensure that he's getting enough protein, Adam starts incorporating vegan protein powders and supplements into his routine. He also makes sure to eat plenty of foods that are naturally high in protein, like beans, nuts, and quinoa. And he gets creative with his snacks, opting for things like roasted chickpeas or almond butter on rice cakes instead of traditional protein bars or shakes.

To maintain his muscle mass, Adam continues to work hard in the gym. He lifts weights regularly but also incorporates more bodyweight exercises, like push-ups and pull-ups, into his routine. He also makes sure to stretch and foam roll regularly to prevent injury and promote recovery.

And it's not just his physical health that improves - Adam also starts to notice a difference in his mental clarity and energy levels. He feels more focused on the field, and he's able to sustain his energy throughout long practices and games without feeling fatigued.

In the end, Adam realizes that going vegan was the right choice for him both personally and professionally. With the help of his dietitian and some careful planning, he's been able to maintain his muscle mass, recover more quickly, and continue performing at the top of his game. And he knows that by choosing a plant-based diet, he's not only taking care of himself but also contributing to a more sustainable and compassionate world.

If you could relate to Adam and his concerns – look carefully at the steps he took until he championed a vegan diet that works for him as well as the environment. There are many stories like that of Adam's – most times it is all about taking the first step and putting your skepticism to the test.

Let's look at some of the common concerns and misconceptions about veganism that can prevent people from adopting this lifestyle or even considering it as an option. Some of the most prevalent ones include:

1. **Lack of protein:** Many people believe that a vegan diet is deficient in protein and that it is impossible to meet the recommended daily intake without consuming animal products. However, this is a myth; there are plenty of plant-based sources of protein, such as beans, lentils, tofu, tempeh, nuts, seeds, and whole grains.

2. **Limited food options:** Some individuals think that being vegan means eating a boring and restricted diet, and that they will have to give up their favorite foods. However, this is not true; there are countless delicious and satisfying vegan recipes that can be enjoyed, ranging from hearty stews and soups to savory burgers and pizzas.

3. **Nutrient deficiencies:** Another misconception is that a vegan diet lacks essential nutrients such as calcium, iron, and vitamin B12. While it is true that some of these nutrients are harder to obtain from plant-based sources, it is possible to meet their requirements by consuming fortified foods and supplements.

4. **Costliness:** Some people believe that eating a vegan diet is expensive, and that they will have to spend a lot of money on specialty products and ingredients. However, this is

not necessarily the case; many plant-based staples, such as rice, beans, and vegetables, are affordable and widely available.

5. **Social isolation:** Some individuals feel that being vegan will make them stand out or be excluded from social events, such as dinners or parties. While it is true that some situations may require some extra planning and communication, like with any dietary restriction, it is possible to enjoy social events and gatherings as a vegan.

6. **All-or-nothing lifestyle**: Some people believe that veganism is an all-or-nothing lifestyle and that you must give up all animal products at once. However, many people transition to veganism gradually, and there are also options for those who want to eat a primarily plant-based diet while still occasionally consuming animal products.

7. **Veganism is only for the wealthy:** Finally, it is a common impression that veganism is only for elite or for people who have lots of free time to cook and prepare their own food. However, there are plenty of affordable, convenient vegan options available in grocery stores and restaurants, and many vegan recipes can be prepared quickly and easily.

Emotional and Physical Changes - What to Expect?

Let's face the truth: Transitioning to a vegan diet can bring about a few changes, both physical and mental. Here are a few things you may experience during the transition:

Changes in digestion:

When you shift from a primarily animal-based diet to a plant-based one, your body will need time to adapt. You may experience some digestive discomfort, such as bloating or gas, as your body adjusts to the new types of foods you are consuming.

Increased energy:

Many people report feeling more energized and alert after switching to a vegan diet. This may be since plant-based diets tend to be higher in complex carbohydrates and fiber, which provide sustained energy throughout the day.

Weight loss:

If you are transitioning to a vegan diet from a high-fat, high-calorie diet, you may notice some weight loss in the first few weeks. This is because plant-based diets tend to be lower in calories and fat than animal-based diets.

Improved skin health:

Some people report clearer, more radiant skin after switching to a vegan diet. This may be because plant-based diets are typically higher in antioxidants and other nutrients that support skin health.

Increased empathy:

For many people, transitioning to a vegan diet is not just about improving their own health, but about reducing their impact on the environment and reducing animal suffering. As a result, many people report feeling more empathy and connection with all living beings.

When transitioning to a vegan diet, it can be common to rely heavily on starchy foods such as French fries, pasta, and rice as they are often viewed as familiar and filling options. However, it's important to remember that while these foods can be a part of a healthy vegan diet, it's important to choose whole grain options and balance them with a variety of other nutrient-dense foods such as fruits, vegetables, legumes, nuts, and seeds.

Consuming a diverse range of plant-based foods ensures that you are getting all the necessary nutrients for optimal health, including protein, fiber, vitamins, and minerals. Additionally, incorporating physical activity into your daily routine can also help support a healthy transition to a vegan diet.

Overall, the transition to a vegan diet can bring about a wide range of positive changes, both for your own health and for the world around you. However, it's important to approach the transition mindfully and make sure you are getting all the necessary nutrients to support optimal health. When you move into this transition with a clear head, better understanding, and some preparation as well as expectations – the journey ahead won't be half as daunting as it may seem in the beginning.

CHAPTER 4:
FUELING YOUR BODY WITH VEGAN NUTRITION

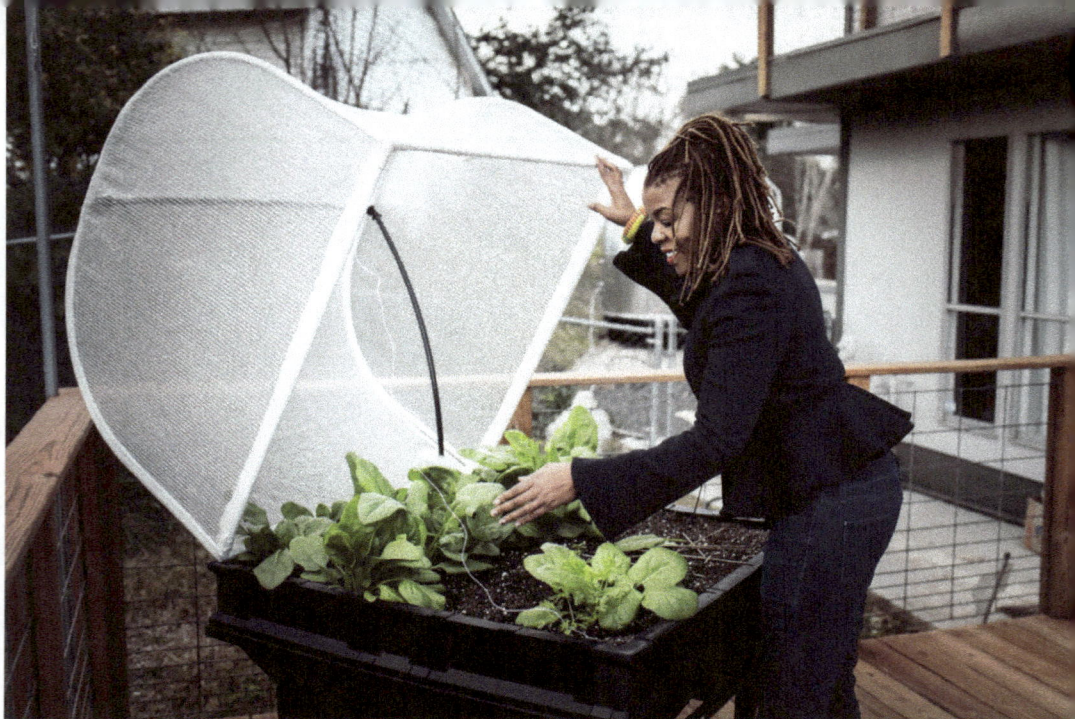

Eating a vegan diet can provide all the necessary nutrients for good health, but it's important to plan your meals carefully to ensure that you're getting enough protein, iron, calcium, and other essential nutrients. You need to understand that plant-based foods now must perform double the work of fulfilling all your nutritional requirements. Here are some tips for getting adequate nutrition on a vegan diet:

Protein: Good sources of plant-based protein include legumes (such as beans, lentils, and peas), nuts and seeds, tofu, tempeh, and seitan.

As a vegan, it's possible to meet your daily protein needs through a well-planned diet. Some good sources of protein for vegans include:

1. Legumes such as lentils, chickpeas, and black beans
2. Soy products such as tofu, tempeh, and edamame
3. Nuts and seeds like almonds, peanuts, and chia seeds

4. Whole grains such as quinoa, brown rice, and oats

The amount of protein that you need will depend on several factors including your age, gender, body weight, and activity level. However, a general guideline is to aim for approximately 0.8 grams of protein per kilogram of body weight per day.

It's also important to note that while plant-based proteins are great for overall health, they may not always contain all the essential amino acids that the body needs. To ensure that you are getting all the necessary amino acids, it's important to eat a variety of protein sources throughout the day.

By incorporating a variety of protein-rich plant-based foods into your diet throughout the day, you can easily meet your daily protein needs as a vegan. It may also be helpful to consult with a registered dietitian to ensure that your diet meets all your nutritional needs.

Iron: Plant-based sources of iron include leafy greens (such as spinach and kale), legumes, whole grains, and fortified cereals and breads.

The most important element of our blood - iron is an essential mineral that plays a crucial role in the human body, including the production of hemoglobin, which carries oxygen to our cells. While animal products are often touted as the best sources of iron, there are plenty of plant-based sources of this important nutrient as well.

Some good sources of iron for vegans include:

1. Legumes such as lentils, chickpeas, and kidney beans
2. Dark leafy greens such as spinach, kale, and collard greens
3. Fortified breakfast cereals and breads
4. Dried fruits such as apricots, prunes, and raisins
5. Nuts and seeds like pumpkin seeds, cashews, and almonds

It's worth noting that non-heme iron, which is the type of iron found in plant-based foods, is not as easily absorbed by the body as heme iron, which is found in animal products. However, there are a few things you can do to help increase absorption of non-heme iron:

- Pair iron-rich foods with vitamin C-rich foods such as citrus fruits, peppers, or broccoli.
- Avoid consuming foods that can interfere with iron absorption, such as calcium-rich foods or tea and coffee.
- Cook in cast-iron cookware, which can help increase the amount of iron in your food.

If you are concerned about your iron intake, particularly if you have a medical condition that affects iron levels, it's worth consulting with a registered dietitian to ensure that you are getting adequate amounts of this important nutrient.

Calcium: Calcium is abundant in many plant-based foods, including leafy greens, tofu made with calcium sulfate, calcium-fortified plant milks and juices, and some legumes.

There are several vegan sources of calcium that can help support bone health. Leafy greens such as kale, collard greens, and bok choy are excellent sources of calcium, as are some fortified plant milks and juices. Tofu that is made with calcium sulfate is also a good source of this important nutrient. Additionally, certain legumes like white beans and chickpeas contain significant amounts of calcium. It's important to include a variety of these foods in your diet to ensure adequate calcium intake, especially if you are following a vegan lifestyle.

Vitamin B12: This nutrient is crucial for vegans because it's only found naturally in animal products. You can get it from supplements or fortified foods like plant milks, breakfast cereals, and nutritional yeast.

Vitamin B12 is an essential nutrient that plays a key role in nerve function and the production of red blood cells. While it's commonly found in animal products, vegans can get their daily requirement of vitamin B12 from fortified foods like plant-based milks, cereals, and nutritional yeast. These fortified products are made by adding B12 to the food during the production process, making them a reliable source of this important nutrient for vegans.

Additionally, some vegan-friendly supplements are available in the form of pills, drops or sprays. It's important for vegans to make sure they consume enough B12 to avoid deficiency, which can lead to anemia, nerve damage and other health issues.

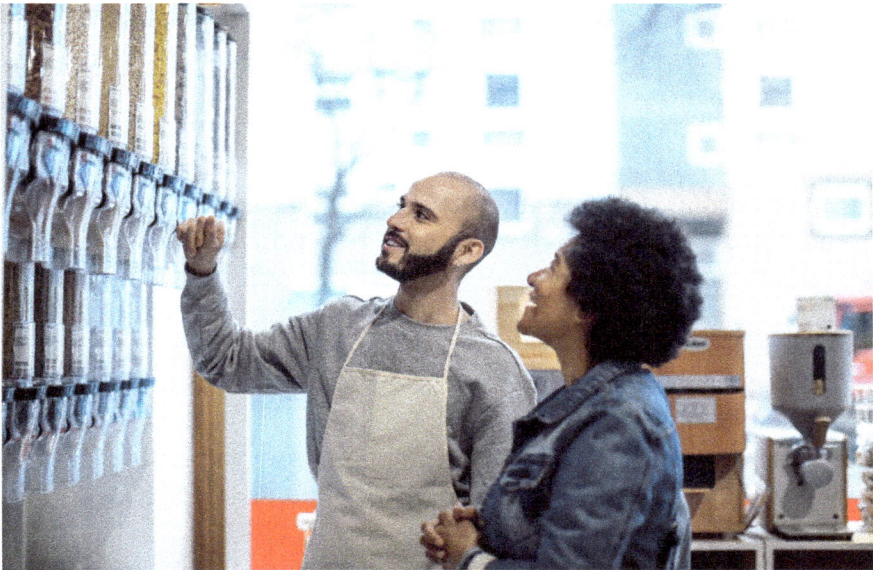

Omega-3 fats: These are important for heart and brain health. Vegan sources include flaxseeds, chia seeds, hemp seeds, walnuts, and algae-based supplements.

While omega 3, 6, and 9 fatty acids are important for overall health, it's important to note that they are not all created equal. Omega-3 fatty acids are essential fatty acids that our bodies cannot produce on their own and therefore need to be obtained through diet. Good sources of omega-3s for vegans include chia seeds, flaxseeds, hemp seeds, walnuts, seaweed, and algae-based supplements.

Omega-6 fatty acids are also essential, but it's easy to get too much of them in the modern Western diet. Many vegans already consume plenty of omega-6s through nuts, seeds, and vegetable oils. However, it's important to maintain a balance between omega-6 and omega-3 intake as excessive amounts of omega-6 can lead to inflammation and other health issues.

Omega-9s are non-essential, meaning that our bodies can produce them on their own. However, they can still be beneficial for heart health and may help lower cholesterol levels. Good sources of omega-9s for vegans include olive oil, avocado, nuts, and seeds.

Vitamin D: This is an essential nutrient that plays a vital role in maintaining bone health, promoting immune function, and regulating mood. While it's most associated with sun exposure, it can also be obtained through diet or supplementation.

As a vegan, some good food sources of vitamin D include fortified plant-based milks or yogurts, mushrooms exposed to UV light, and fortified breakfast cereals. However, it can be difficult to obtain enough vitamin D from food alone, especially during the winter months when sun exposure may be limited.

If you are unable to obtain sufficient vitamin D through food, it may be necessary to supplement with a vitamin D3 supplement. Vegan-friendly vitamin D3 supplements are available and can be found at most health food stores or online retailers.

Note that vitamin D requirements can vary based on factors such as age, gender, and geographical location. It may be helpful to consult with a healthcare provider or registered dietitian to determine the appropriate dosage and source of vitamin D for your individual needs.

It's important to eat a varied and balanced diet that includes plenty of whole foods, fruits and vegetables, and healthy sources of protein, carbohydrates, and fat to support optimal health.

Bonus Tips: The Lesser-known Plant Based foods.

When I first discovered these, I was amazed. We usually only get to see and read about the same old basic plant-based foods, but these lesser-known ones can provide unique health benefits and add variety to a vegan diet. Here are a few examples:

1. **Seaweed:** Seaweed is an excellent source of iodine, which is important for thyroid function. It is also high in minerals such as calcium, iron, and magnesium. Packs a punch in terms of flavor too!

2. **Tempeh:** Tempeh is a fermented soy product that is high in protein and probiotics, which can help support gut health. I know I have mentioned it above a bunch of times – but somehow most people are unaware of this great protein option.

3. **Jackfruit:** Jackfruit is a versatile fruit that can be used as a meat substitute in dishes such as tacos and BBQ sandwiches. It is high in fiber, vitamin C, and potassium. Its texture is so eerily like meat, you will find it hard to tell.

4. **Amaranth:** Amaranth is a gluten-free grain that is high in protein, fiber, and iron. It has a nutty flavor and can be used in place of rice or quinoa. Perfect for days when you feel bored of the two basic staples.

5. **Nutritional yeast:** Nutritional yeast is a deactivated form of yeast that is often used as a seasoning or cheese substitute. It is high in protein and B vitamins, including vita-

min B12, which is important for vegans. (Did someone say cheese?)

All in all, incorporating a variety of plant-based foods into your diet can help ensure that you are getting all the necessary nutrients for optimal health. Experimenting with different flavors and textures can also make meals more enjoyable and exciting.

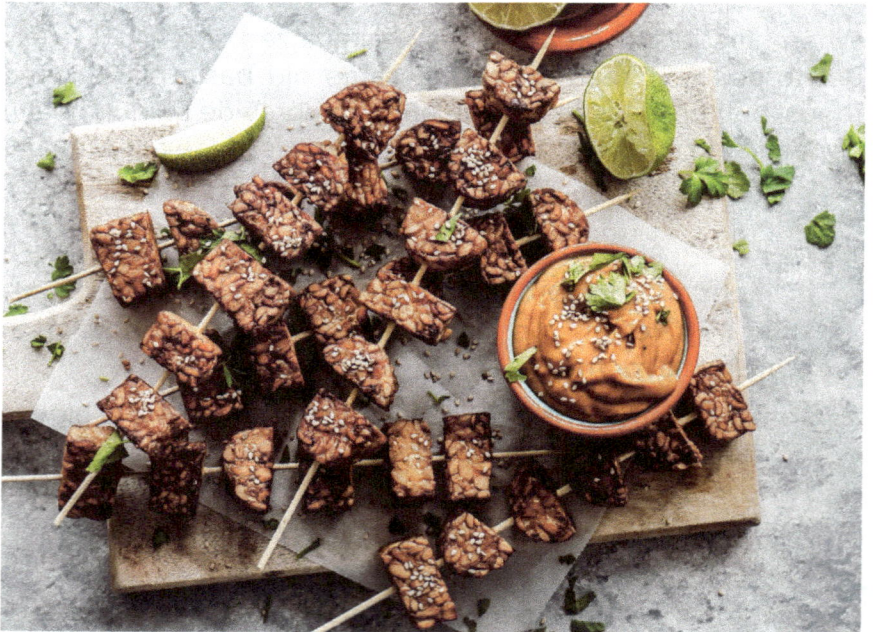

CHAPTER 5:
SOY THE CONTROVERSIAL VEGAN FOOD

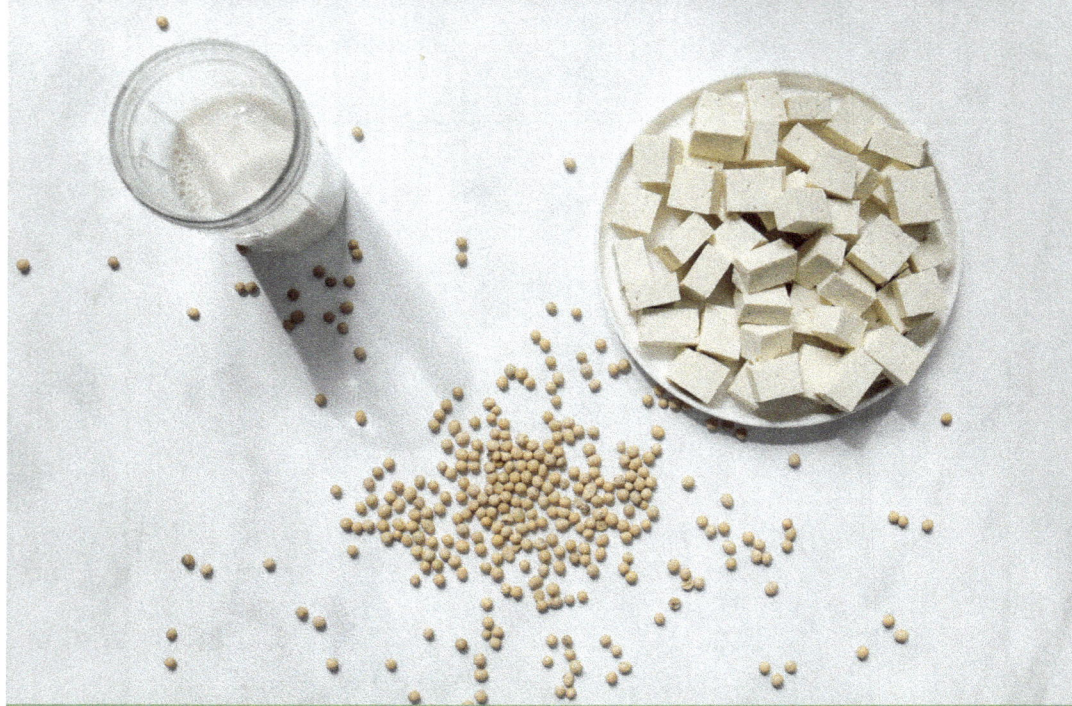

Soy has been associated with many myths and misconceptions, which is why I decided to give this special attention through a separately dedicated chapter.

Soy is a type of legume that is often used in food products such as tofu, soy milk, and soy sauce. It is grown in many parts of the world and is a staple crop in many Asian countries. Soybeans, the source of soy, are originally from East Asia and have been cultivated for thousands of years. Today, soybeans are grown in many countries around the world, including the United States, Brazil, Argentina, and China. Soy is a versatile food ingredient and is used in a variety of products.

To make soy products, soybeans are first cleaned and soaked in water. They are then ground into a fine paste, which is mixed with water and boiled to create soy milk. The soy milk can be used as is, or it can be further processed to make other products such as tofu or tempeh.

In the case of tofu, soy milk is coagulated using a substance such as calcium sulfate to create curds. The curds are then pressed, resulting in a firm tofu product. Tempeh, on the other hand, is made by allowing the soybeans to ferment and bind together into a dense cake.

There are a few myths surrounding soy, with one of the most common being that it can increase the risk of breast cancer. However, there is no scientific evidence to support this claim. Soy is a beneficial part of a healthy diet and contains essential nutrients such as protein and fiber. It can also have positive effects on heart health and may even reduce the risk of certain types of cancer. It's important to consume soy in moderation and choose whole soy foods such as tofu, edamame, or soy milk instead of highly processed products.

Another common myth surrounding soy is that it can negatively affect male hormones and fertility. However, studies have shown that soy intake in moderate amounts does not impact male hormone levels or fertility. Another myth is that soy is not good for thyroid health, but again, scientific evidence shows that moderate amounts of soy consumption do not interfere with thyroid function in healthy individuals.

Overall, soy is a nutritious and beneficial part of a healthy diet when consumed in moderation and whole food forms. It's important to differentiate between myths and actual scientific evidence when making dietary choices.

There are some myths surrounding soy consumption that may lead some people to believe it is bad for them. These myths may have been perpetuated due to a lack of scientific evidence or misinformation.

One common myth of such nature is that soy contains phytoestrogens that can mimic the effects of estrogen in the body, leading to hormonal imbalances and potential health issues. However, studies have shown that moderate levels of soy consumption do not have significant effects on hormone levels or reproductive health.

It's important to note that like many other foods, soy should be consumed in moderation as part of a healthy balanced diet. It's always best to consult with a healthcare professional or registered dietitian if you have any concerns about your dietary habits.

You can find ample scientific studies on the effects of soy consumption by searching reputable sources such as PubMed, which is a database of biomedical research articles. Additionally, many health organizations such as the American Heart Association, American Cancer Society, and Academy of Nutrition and Dietetics have published statements or guidelines on the role of soy in a healthy diet, which are based on scientific evidence. It's always important to critically evaluate any source of information and ensure that it is from a credible and trustworthy source.

There is no conclusive evidence that soy is bad for most people. Research suggests that soy consumption can have health benefits such as lowering cholesterol levels and reducing the risk of certain cancers. However, some individuals may have allergies or intolerances to soy, and there are concerns about the impact of soy farming on the environment. It's always important to consult with a healthcare professional before making any significant changes to your diet.

Tofu is another target. And no, tofu is not inherently bad. It can be a nutritious and versatile ingredient in a balanced diet. Tofu is made from soy milk and is a good source of protein, calcium, and iron. However, as with any food, the way tofu is prepared and consumed can impact its healthfulness. For example, fried or heavily processed tofu may be higher in calories and unhealthy fats. It's important to consider portion sizes and preparation methods when including tofu in your diet.

There are many healthy ways to incorporate tofu into your diet. Here are a few ideas:

- Crumble or slice tofu and add it to stir-fries, soups, and salads for a protein boost.
- Blend tofu with fruit and almond milk for a creamy, high-protein smoothie.
- Use silken tofu as a base for dips and spreads, such as hummus or guacamole.
- Grill or bake tofu and add it to sandwiches and wraps.
- Use tofu as a substitute for eggs in vegan quiches and frittatas.

Like anything, Soy can be over-processed when it undergoes extensive heating, refining, and extraction methods. This can remove many of the nutrients and beneficial compounds found in the original soybean, leaving behind a highly processed product that may not have the same health benefits.

Additionally, highly processed soy products may contain additives, preservatives, and other ingredients that are not necessarily beneficial for our health. It's important to look for minimally processed soy products, such as tofu, tempeh, and edamame when incorporating soy into your diet.

Studies have shown that incorporating whole soy foods into your diet can have a positive impact on reducing the risk for certain chronic diseases. Soybeans are a good source of protein, fiber, and various vitamins and minerals. They also contain isoflavones, which are plant compounds that have been found to have potential health benefits.

Research suggests that regularly consuming whole soy foods such as tofu, edamame, soy milk, and miso may reduce the risk of heart disease, diabetes, and certain types of cancer. However, it's important to note that soy foods should not be relied upon as the sole treatment or prevention method for these diseases and should be consumed as part of an overall healthy diet.

It's worth noting that soy can also be over-processed when it is genetically modified or grown with pesticides and other chemicals. To avoid these potential health risks, it's best to choose organic, non-GMO soy products whenever possible. And as with any food, moderation is key - while soy can be a healthy addition to a balanced diet, consuming too much soy may have negative effects on hormone levels and overall health. It's important to listen to your body and make choices that work best for you.

CHAPTER 6:
GMO'S AND WHAT IS IT?

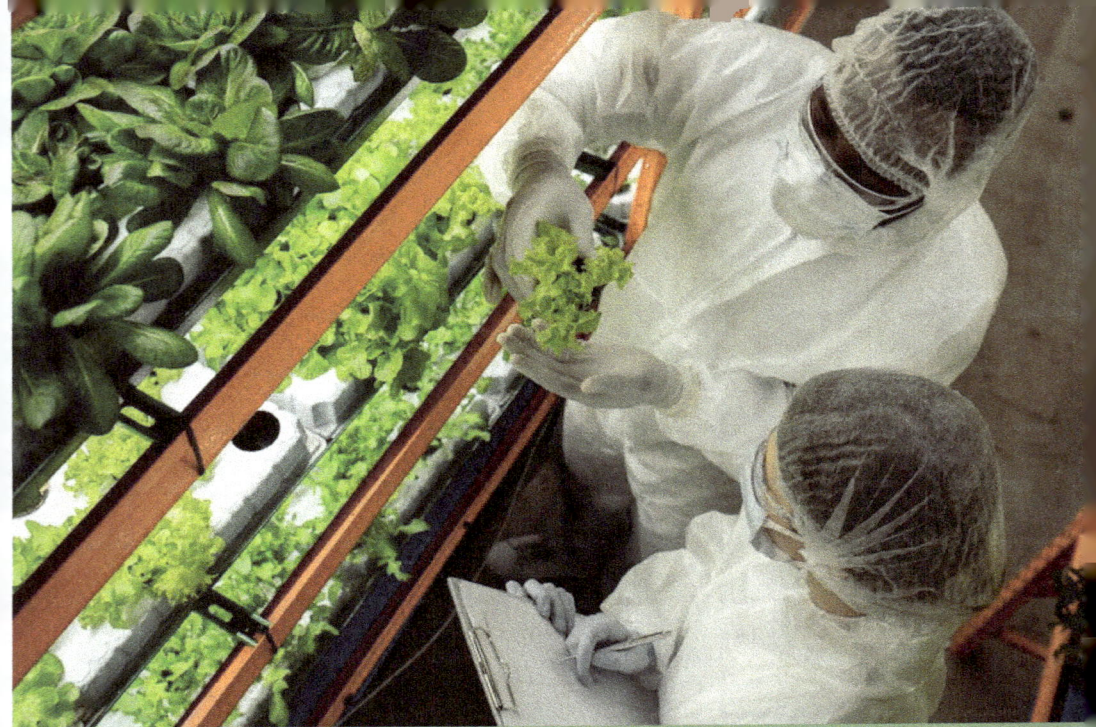

GMOs, or Genetically Modified Organisms, are organisms whose genetic material has been artificially altered through genetic engineering. This process involves the insertion of genes from one organism into another to create a desired trait, such as resistance to pests or herbicides. Non-GMOs, on the other hand, are organisms that have not been genetically modified in this way and have been grown using traditional farming methods.

Non-GMO products are typically thought to be free from potential health and environmental risks associated with GMOs.

Some examples of organic, non-GMO soy products include tofu, tempeh, edamame, and soy milk made from whole, organic soybeans. It's important to look for products that are certified organic and non-GMO to ensure that they meet these standards. Additionally, you can look for labels such as the USDA Organic seal and the Non-GMO Project Verified seal to further confirm the product's authenticity.

Scientists conduct rigorous testing and evaluation of genetically modified organisms to ensure their safety for human consumption and the environment. This includes examining the potential impacts on human health, biodiversity, and ecosystems. Regulatory agencies such as the US Food and Drug Administration (FDA), the European Food Safety Authority (EFSA), and the World Health Organization (WHO) oversee the approval process for GMOs and require extensive testing and documentation before a GMO product can be approved for use.

Additionally, many scientific studies are conducted to evaluate the long-term effects of GMOs on both humans and the environment. However, there is still ongoing debate and controversy surrounding the safety of using GMOs in agriculture and food production.

However, there are several potential benefits to using GMOs in agriculture and food production. For example, GMO crops can be engineered to be more resistant to pests, diseases, and environmental stressors, which can increase crop yields and reduce the need for chemical pesticides and herbicides. This can also lead to more sustainable farming practices by reducing the environmental impact of agricultural practices.

Additionally, GMOs can also be engineered to have improved nutrition, taste, and texture, which can lead to more appealing and nutritious food products. Overall, the use of GMOs in agriculture and food production has the potential to increase food security, improve crop yields, and reduce the environmental impact of farming practices.

There are many other organic and non-GMO food products to look out for! Some examples include fruits and vegetables, grains (such as rice, quinoa, and oats), dairy products, eggs, meat, and poultry. It's important to read labels carefully and look for certifications such as the USDA Organic seal and Non-GMO Project Verified seal to ensure that the product meets these standards. Additionally, buying locally grown produce from farmers' markets or joining a CSA can help ensure that your food is fresh, organic, and non-GMO.

To identify organic and non-GMO products in the grocery store, consumers can look for labels such as the USDA Organic seal and the Non-GMO Project Verified seal. These labels indicate that the product meets certain standards and has been verified by a third party. Additionally, some stores may have specific sections or displays for organic and non-GMO products, so it's important to explore the store and ask questions if you're unsure. Reading labels carefully and researching brands can also help you make informed choices about the products you buy.

Some examples of GMO foods include genetically modified corn, soybeans, canola, sugar beets, papaya, and cottonseed. Other common GMO ingredients include corn syrup, high fructose corn syrup, and soy lecithin. It's important to note that many processed foods contain ingredients derived from GMO crops, so it's often difficult to avoid GMOs entirely if you consume a lot of packaged or processed foods.

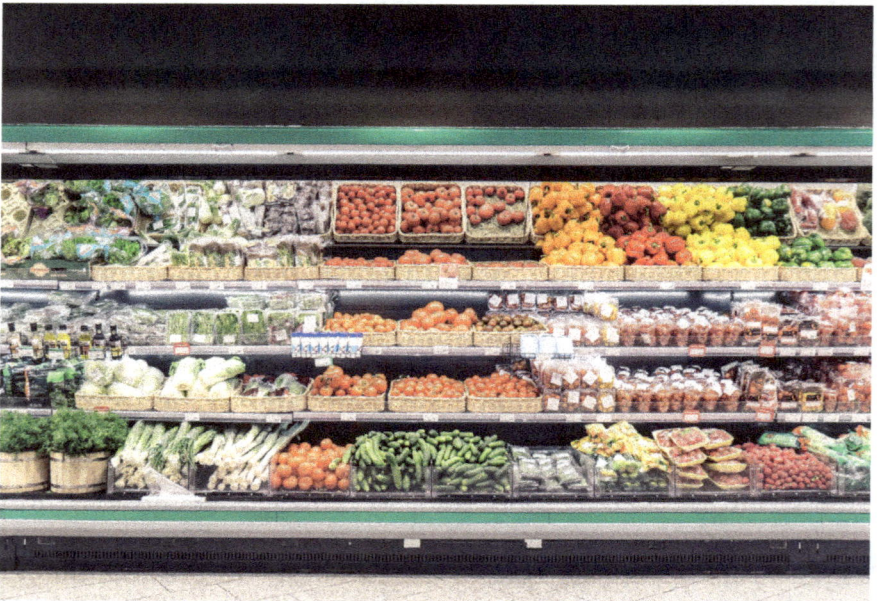

There are many different types of GMO foods, here are 50 common examples:

1. Corn
2. Soybeans
3. Canola
4. Sugar beets
5. Papaya
6. Cottonseed
7. Alfalfa
8. Squash
9. Tomatoes
10. Potatoes
11. Apples
12. Rice
13. Flax
14. Wheat
15. Barley
16. Sweet peppers
17. Cucumbers
18. Zucchini
19. Carrots
20. Onions
21. Garlic
22. Celery
23. Broccoli
24. Cauliflower
25. Spinach
26. Lettuce
27. Kale
28. Radishes
29. Beets
30. Peas
31. Lentils
32. Chickpeas
33. Sorghum
34. Sugar cane
35. Sunflower
36. Rapeseed
37. Mustard
38. Fava beans
39. Peanuts
40. Hazelnuts
41. Almonds
42. Walnuts
43. Pistachios
44. Cashews
45. Macadamia nuts
46. Coconut
47. Pineapple
48. Mango
49. Grapefruit
50. Lemons

GMOs can have nutritional value depending on the traits that have been introduced or modified. For example, some GMO crops are engineered to contain higher levels of certain vitamins or nutrients, while others may be more resistant to pests or diseases, which can increase their yield and availability. However, there is ongoing debate and research into the potential long-term effects of consuming GMO foods on human health.

CHAPTER 7:
COOKING WITH OILS

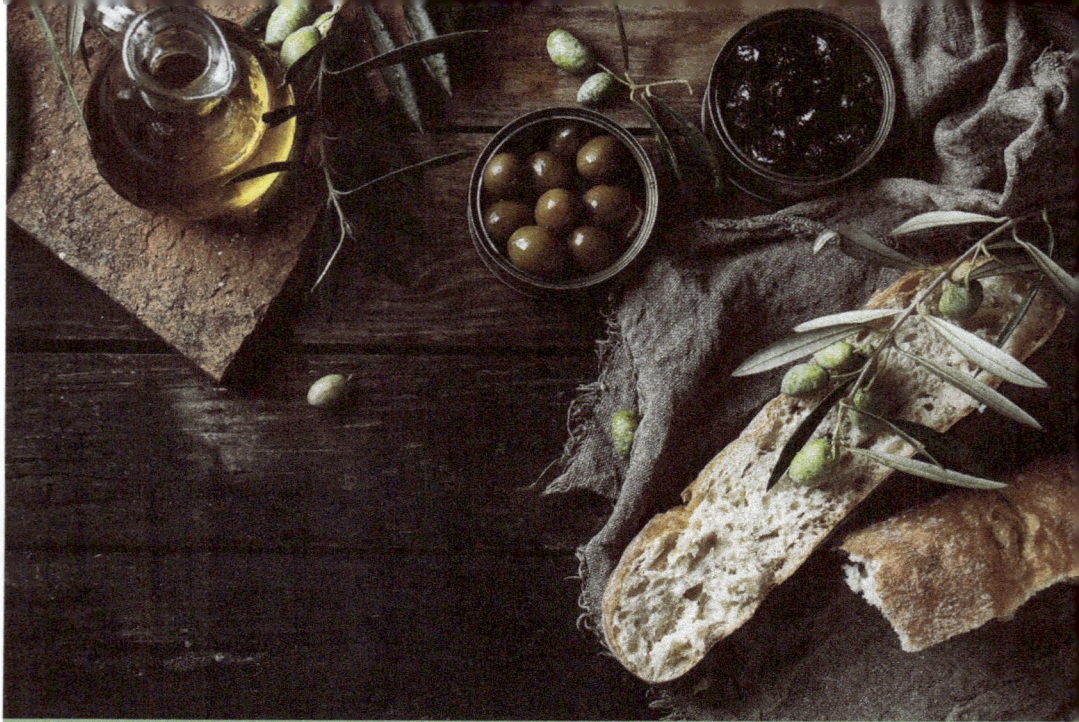

Let's face it — when it comes to cooking our own vegan meals — the need for some form of fat or grease to cook with is, inevitable. Based on years of research coupled with lots of trying and testing — here is a list of cooking oils that are great for vegan cooking and provide excellent nutritional value.

1. **Avocado oil**

   You might be discouraged by the pricing of avocado oil, but you also need to remember that health perks are worth the few extra dollars. Luckily, there are different sizes of avocado oil bottles that are available for affordable prices.

   One of the properties of avocado oil that makes it ideal for vegan dishes is its high smoke-point. Furthermore, avocado oil allows you to prepare vegetables, make salad dressings, bake, and, most importantly, you will get a vitamin E supplementation, which comes as an antioxidant.

2. **Coconut oil**

   Coconut oil is another popular oil choice that's preferred by many people, especially those who stick to a vegan diet. One of the properties that makes coconut oil good is the fact that it contains saturated fatty acid, which is responsible for enhancing its stability to heat.

   The oil is also a perfect immunity-boosting solution, and for those who don't want to keep oils in the refrigerator, this is a good choice because coconut oil is not affected by oxidation.

3. **Light olive oil**

   Even used by a lot of non-vegans, olive oil is a unique oil for a vegan diet because it is among few that are extracted by some fruit. The oil contains a large amount of healthy and flavorful compounds that include volatile aromatic elements such as esters and terpenes; pigments such as chlorophyll; and several antioxidants, including phenolic compounds and carotenoids.

   The process of making olive oil includes taking almost-ripe olives and grinding them to form a paste, which is then allowed to stay untouched for the oil to squeeze out. The first extraction is what is referred to as "extra virgin oil." Like many healthy oils for vegan meals, olive oil contains a high amount of monounsaturated fats and a low amount of saturated and polyunsaturated fats, making it a stable choice for a vegan diet.

4. **Rice-bran oil**

   A rather new one and unheard of - rice bran is extracted from the germ (or husk) of rice and can be extracted using solvent extraction or pressing done in an expeller. After extraction, the oil is ready for use, as there is no need for refining because at this stage it is considered refined and ready for use.

Some of the benefits of bran oil include a high smoke point, which is beneficial when you are using it in high-heat applications such as frying. Health reports have also confirmed that the fat profile of bran is optimal, making it a healthy choice. Additionally, rice-bran oil contains chemicals such as tocotrienols, which are believed to possess antioxidant properties.

5. **Canola oil**

   Now here is one that you must have heard of before and even used. Canola oil was first developed in the 1970s after it was discovered from a plant that belongs to the mustard family. The plant underwent selective breeding to help improve the quality of the oil, and today it is among the most preferred oils for vegan dishes.

   Some of the unique features of the oil include a high composition of monounsaturated fats, a low percentage of saturated fats, and the fact that it contains a neutral flavor thanks to low amounts of erucic acid.

   Even when unrefined, canola oil exhibits a high smoking point, which makes it an ideal choice for meals that require heating to high temperatures. Canola oil also contains a large proportion of omega-3 fatty acids, which are good for the health of the consumer.

There is some debate around the health effects of canola oil. Canola oil is a type of vegetable oil made from the rapeseed plant, and it's often used in cooking and baking.

On one hand, canola oil is high in monounsaturated fats, which have been shown to have positive effects on heart health. It's also low in saturated fat and cholesterol.

However, some studies have suggested that canola oil may have negative effects on inflammation and oxidative stress in the body. There have also been concerns about the use of genetically modified rapeseed plants in the production of canola oil.

Overall, it's important to consider the potential risks and benefits of canola oil, and to choose high-quality sources of fats in your diet. Alternatives to canola oil include olive oil, avocado oil, and coconut oil. As with any dietary choices, it's best to you know with a healthcare provider or registered dietitian for personalized advice.

Canola oil is generally considered safe for cooking, as it has a high smoke point and can withstand high temperatures without breaking down or producing harmful compounds. However, it's important to use canola oil in moderation and to avoid using it for deep frying, as this can cause the oil to break down and produce unhealthy compounds.

Additionally, it's important to choose high-quality sources of canola oil, as some low-quality oils may be mixed with other types of oils or contain harmful additives. It's best to look for organic, non-GMO canola oil that is cold-pressed or expeller-pressed, as these methods preserve the natural nutrients and flavors of the oil.

6. **Safflower Oil**

   Safflower oil presents a neutral taste great for marinades, dips and sauces as well as lightly searing and sauteing on the stovetop. Like avocado oil, it has a high smoke point (around 510 degrees) and it's high in unsaturated fatty acids.

   A recent study found that incorporating this healthy oil into your diet can help reduce the risk of coronary heart disease and improve inflammation, blood sugar management and cholesterol.

7. **Grapeseed Oil**

   Grapeseed oil is rich in omega-6 fatty acids and vitamin E. By incorporating this heart-friendly oil into your diet, you can enjoy a reduced risk of heart disease because of its high antioxidant properties. Try using it for stir-frying, sauteing and searing vegetables and protein.

8. **Sesame Oil**

   Sesame oil has a lower smoke point than the others, but it still should be added to your list of heart-healthy oils. It's high in sesamol and sesaminol, which are antioxidants shown to reduce heart cell damage.

   You can use sesame oil to sauté your favorite vegetables, as a salad dressing ingredient and most general-purpose cooking. The flavor profile is more intense and nuttier than the other oils, so keep that in mind when cooking.

What Makes Oil Healthy?

To ensure that you are purchasing high-quality oils and free of harmful additives, it's important to look for certain indicators on the label. Here are a few things to keep in mind:

1. **Organic:** Look for organic canola oil, which is free of pesticides and other harmful chemicals.
2. **Non-GMO:** Choose non-GMO canola oil, which means it was made from non-genetically modified plants.
3. **Cold-pressed or expeller-pressed:** These methods of extraction preserve the natural nutrients and flavors of the oil.
4. **High smoke point:** Make sure the oil has a high smoke point, which means it can withstand high temperatures without breaking down.
5. **No additives:** Check the label for any added preservatives, flavors, or colors, which can be harmful to your health.

By paying attention to these factors, you can ensure that you are buying high-quality canola oil that is free of harmful additives.

Whether you're sautéing up some veggies for a stir fry or browning a piece of fish, it's important to also consider the smoke point of your oil. The smoke point refers to the temperature at which it starts to burn and smoke. When oil reaches that temperature and you consume it, not only do you receive an unpleasant burnt taste, but you also destroy beneficial nutrients. Below are five heart-healthy cooking oils that tolerate high heat cooking.

Some of the best oils to cook with are those that have a high smoke point and are low in saturated and trans fats. Some examples include:

1. **Olive oil** - This oil is high in monounsaturated fats and has a medium smoke point, making it suitable for cooking at medium temperatures.
2. **Avocado oil** - This oil is high in monounsaturated fats and has a high smoke point, making it suitable for cooking at high temperatures.
3. **Canola oil** - As mentioned earlier, this oil is versatile and can be used for cooking at low to medium temperatures.
4. **Peanut oil** - This oil has a high smoke point and is often used in Asian cuisine for stir-frying and deep-frying.
5. **Grapeseed oil** - This oil has a high smoke point and is often used in baking and cooking at high temperatures.

All in all, oil is an essential part of many recipes, whether it is used as a dressing, a cooking agent or to add body to a sauce, salsa, or dip, this important ingredient really brings out the flavor in our dishes, making them a sizzling success.

When it comes to cooking oils, there are some that are better for you than others. Oils that are high in unsaturated fats (like olive oil, avocado oil, and canola oil) are healthier options than those that are high in saturated or trans fats (like coconut oil or vegetable shortening).

Unsaturated fats have been shown to help reduce inflammation, lower cholesterol levels, and provide other health benefits. On the other hand, saturated and trans fats have been linked to increased risk of heart disease, stroke, and other chronic health conditions.

Of course, it's important to remember that all oils are still a source of calories and fat, so portion control is key. It's also a good idea to choose oils that are minimally processed and avoid those that are high in additives or preservatives.

CHAPTER 8:
THE EFFECT VEGANISM HAS ON THE ENVIRONMENT

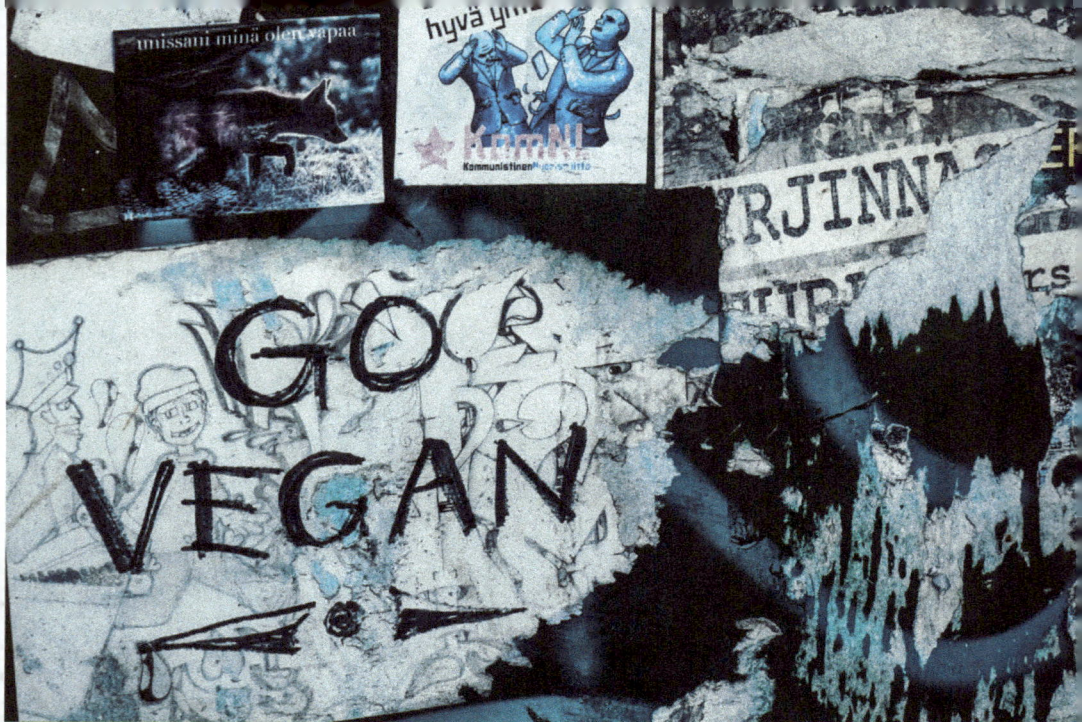

Veganism has become an increasingly popular lifestyle choice in recent years, and for good reason. One major benefit of veganism is its positive impact on the environment. In fact, ever since I adopted this diet – the impact I am making to my planet has been a major motivator in maintaining this lifestyle. In this chapter, I want to explore with you the various ways in which choosing a plant-based lifestyle can help to mitigate environmental damage and promote sustainability.

Firstly, animal agriculture is a significant contributor to greenhouse gas emissions, accounting for around 14.5% of global emissions. The production of animal products such as meat, dairy, and eggs require many resources, including land, water, and feed. This process also produces significant amounts of greenhouse gases, such as methane and carbon dioxide, which contribute to global warming. By reducing the demand for animal products, veganism can help to reduce these harmful emissions and slow down the effects of climate change.

In addition to reducing greenhouse gas emissions, a plant-based lifestyle can also help to preserve biodiversity. The use of land for animal agriculture often involves deforestation and destruction of natural habitats, which can lead to the extinction of certain species. By choosing plant-based foods instead of animal products, individuals can help to protect these endangered species and support the natural ecosystems that they inhabit.

Another important aspect of veganism's impact on the environment is its potential to promote sustainability. By choosing plant-based options, individuals can reduce their overall carbon footprint and contribute to a more sustainable food system.

Let me give you an example. The average American consumes around 100kg of meat per year. A study showed that the production of only 1kg of beef (not even mentioning other types of meats) generates 60kg of greenhouse gas emissions! While a vegan substitute like tofu only generates 3.5kg of the same. Imagine how by switching from beef to tofu – you are reducing your carbon footprint by almost 95%!

This is not all. Veganism can also encourage changes in consumer behavior and attitudes towards food production. As more people adopt veganism, there may be a shift towards more sustainable and environmentally friendly farming practices, such as regenerative agriculture, which can help to mitigate the effects of climate change and promote long-term ecological health.

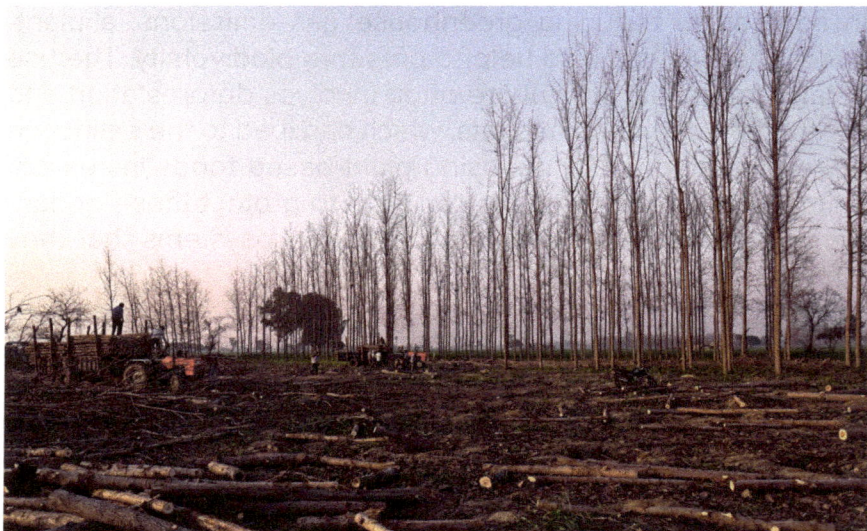

It is no surprise that animal agriculture requires vast amounts of land, water, and energy for production, processing, and transportation. To produce animal products, energy is needed to grow crops for animal feed, transport animals and their feed, operate machinery, and process and package meat, dairy, and eggs. In contrast to that, Plant-based foods require significantly fewer resources to produce than animal products. For example, it takes much less land, water, and fertilizer to grow plants for human consumption than it does to grow crops for animal feed. This means that plant-based foods have a much lower carbon footprint than animal products.

This can inevitably help address the issue of water scarcity. Animal agriculture requires significant amounts of water for both the production of feed and the animals themselves. This can lead to serious water shortages in certain regions, especially those where water resources are already limited. By choosing plant-based foods, individuals can significantly reduce their water usage and contribute to a more sustainable water system.

Animal agriculture is not only responsible for water shortage but also for pollution of whatever little water bodies we are left with. Manure and fertilizer runoff from animal farms can contaminate local waterways, leading to harmful algal blooms, dead zones, and other ecological impacts. By reducing demand for animal

products, we can also reduce the volume of waste produced by these facilities, and thus decrease the risk of water pollution.

Lastly, something I can personally vouch for from experience is that veganism can also have positive impacts on human health. By eliminating animal products from their diet, individuals may experience improved digestion, increased energy levels, and better overall well-being. This can lead to reduced healthcare costs and a healthier population overall, which can have far-reaching benefits for society.

In conclusion, veganism has a significant impact on the environment in many positive ways and the benefits of this lifestyle are far reaching in the preservation of our planet. By reducing greenhouse gas emissions, preserving biodiversity, promoting sustainability, addressing water scarcity, and improving human health, veganism can help to create a more sustainable and equitable future for all. As more people adopt this lifestyle, we can work towards a more environmentally conscious and responsible world.

CHAPTER 9:
ANIMAL TREATMENT IN SOME FACTORY FARMS

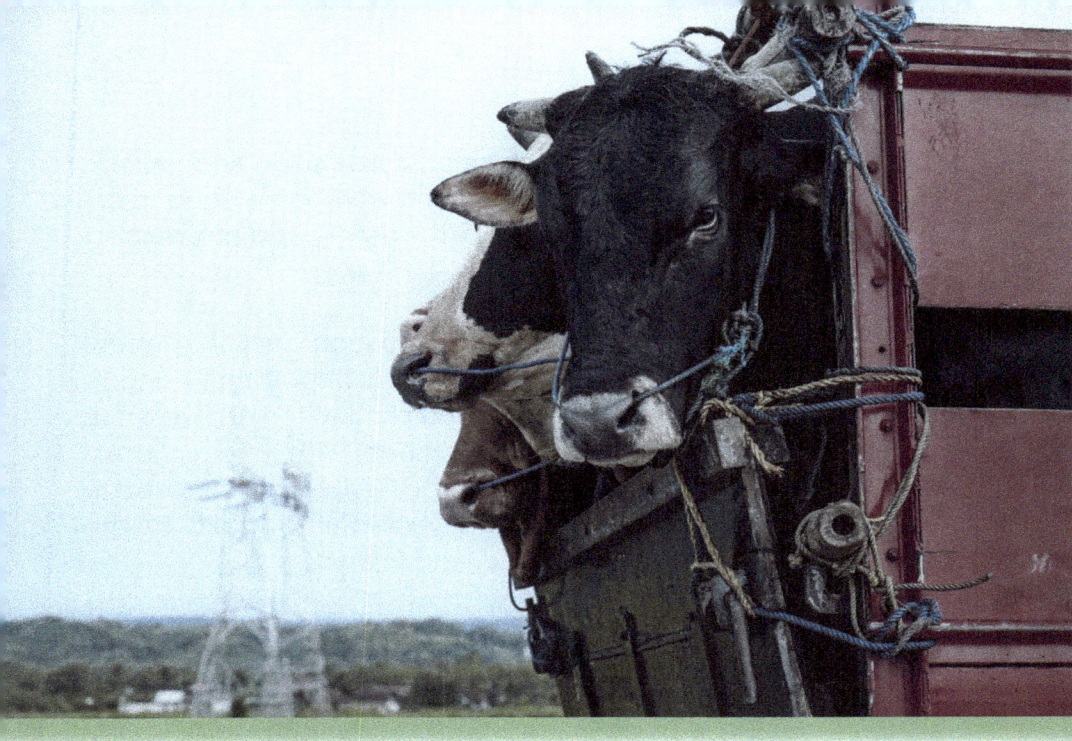

Fair and square, let's now dive deep into the issue that motivates many to adopt veganism. Animal treatment in factory farms is a complex issue that has received increasing attention in recent years. Many animal welfare experts and activists have raised concerns about the living conditions of animals in factory farms, including cramped and unsanitary conditions, lack of access to natural light and fresh air, and overcrowding. These conditions can lead to physical and psychological stress for the animals, which can impact their health and well-being.

Additionally, many factory farms engage in practices such as tail docking, debeaking, and castration without anesthesia, which can cause pain and suffering for the animals. There are also concerns about the use of antibiotics and hormones in animal agriculture, which can contribute to the development of antibiotic-resistant bacteria and potentially harm human health.

Efforts to improve animal welfare in factory farms have included the adoption of animal welfare standards and certification programs by some companies, as well as the promotion of alternative farming methods such as pasture-raised and organic production. However, there is still much work to be done to ensure that animals raised for food are treated with the respect and dignity they deserve.

There is a significant amount of information available about animal welfare in factory farms. Firstly, it is important to understand that most animals used for food production are raised in crowded and often unsanitary conditions, with little to no access to the outdoors or natural environments. This can lead to a range of negative physical and psychological effects on the animals, including stress, disease, and injury.

Furthermore, many factory farms use methods such as confinement, tail docking, castration, and other painful procedures without proper anesthesia or pain relief. This can cause unnecessary suffering for the animals and raises ethical concerns about our treatment of them.

There are also environmental impacts associated with factory farming practices, such as pollution from large-scale manure storage and disposal, greenhouse gas emissions from animal waste and feed production, and depletion of natural resources such as water and land.

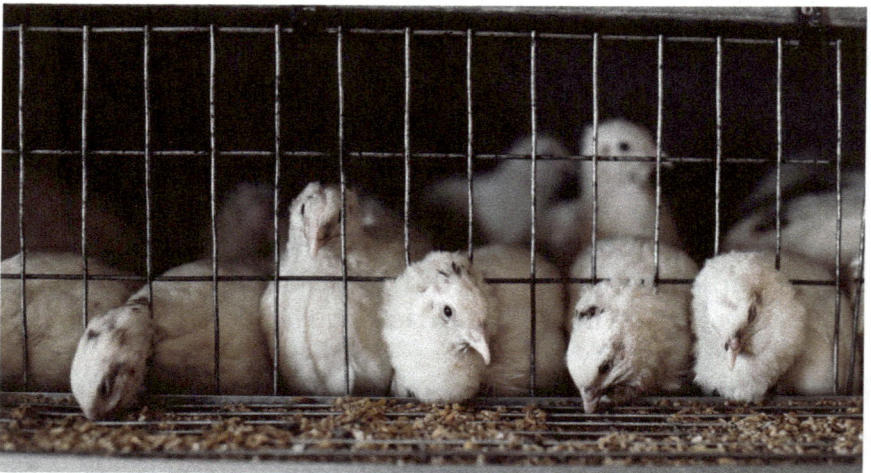

Overall, the topic of animal welfare in factory farms is complex and multifaceted, but it is an important issue to consider in our food choices and agricultural practices.

There have been some noteworthy successes in improving animal welfare standards in factory farms. Some companies have developed animal welfare standards and certification programs that require farmers to meet certain criteria for the care and treatment of their animals. These criteria may include providing adequate space and ventilation, access to clean water and food, and appropriate veterinary care.

In addition, some companies have implemented alternative farming methods such as pasture-raised and organic production which can improve animal welfare by allowing animals more space and opportunities to exhibit natural behaviors.

There have also been legislative efforts to improve conditions for farm animals. In the United States, for example, some states have passed laws requiring larger cages for hens in egg production and banning the use of gestation crates for pigs in pork production.

While progress has been made, there is still much work to be done to ensure that animals raised for food are treated humanely and with respect. It is important for consumers to continue to raise awareness about animal welfare issues and to support companies and legislative efforts that prioritize animal welfare.

Not all is dark and hopeless in this world of hyper-consumerism. I am including some examples of companies that have successfully implemented animal welfare standards and certification programs, below:

Whole Foods Market: This grocery store chain has an animal welfare rating system that rates the welfare of the animals raised for their meat and eggs.

Nestle: This global food company has committed to sourcing from suppliers who meet certain animal welfare standards, including no debeaking of chickens and no tail docking of pigs.

Chipotle: This fast-food chain sources its meat from suppliers who meet its animal welfare standards, which include providing outdoor access and avoiding the use of antibiotics.

Patagonia Provisions: This food company has a certification program called Regenerative Organic Certified, which includes animal welfare standards such as access to the outdoors and humane slaughter.

Costco: This membership-only warehouse club has a commitment to only sourcing cage-free eggs and pork from suppliers who meet certain animal welfare standards.

McDonald's: This fast-food giant has committed to only sourcing cage-free eggs and pork from suppliers who meet certain animal welfare standards. They also have a commitment to sourcing only sustainable fish.

Tyson Foods: This major meat producer has implemented animal welfare audits at all its facilities and has committed to phasing out the use of certain antibiotics in its chicken production.

Certified Humane: This certification program ensures that animals are raised with certain humane treatment standards, including access to outdoor space, proper nutrition, and no confinement crates or cages.

The American Grass-fed Association: This certification program ensures that grass-fed animals are raised with certain standards, such as access to pasture and a diet free of grains and artificial hormones.

These are just a few examples of companies that have taken steps to improve animal welfare in their supply chains. It's important to do research and support companies that prioritize animal welfare if that's important to you.

CHAPTER 10:
CAN I GO VEGAN WHILE PREGNANT?

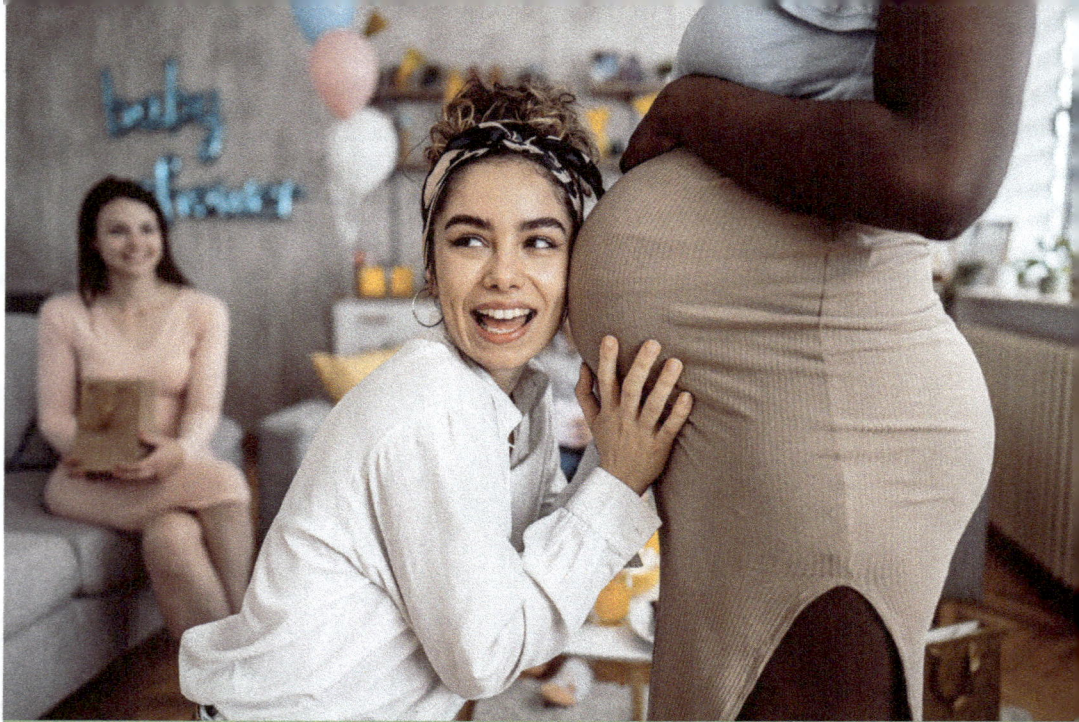

This is a question I have often received from women considering a vegan lifestyle. How to adopt a vegan lifestyle while pregnant and breastfeeding? It's important to note that a well-planned vegan diet can provide all the necessary nutrients for both you and your baby, but it's important to consult with your healthcare provider to ensure that you're meeting your nutritional needs.

Here I have included some of the most essential nutrients and the foods you can find them in during your pregnancy.

Protein:

Protein is an essential nutrient during pregnancy and can be found in a variety of plant-based foods such as beans, lentils, tofu, tempeh, nuts, and seeds. Including a variety of these foods in your diet can help you meet your protein needs.

Iron:

Iron is another important nutrient, especially during pregnancy. Good sources of plant-based iron include leafy greens, tofu, tempeh, legumes, whole grains, seeds, and nuts. It's important to consume vitamin C-rich foods alongside iron-rich foods to enhance absorption.

Calcium:

Calcium is necessary for fetal skeletal development and can be found in fortified plant-based milks, leafy greens, tofu, and calcium-set tofu. Supplements may also be recommended by your healthcare provider.

Omega-3 fatty acids:

Omega-3 fatty acids are important for brain development in the fetus and can be found in flaxseeds, chia seeds, hemp seeds, walnuts, and algae-based supplements.

Vitamin B12:

Vitamin B12 is essential for proper nerve and brain function and can be found in fortified plant-based milks, cereals, and nutritional yeast. Supplements may also be recommended.

In addition to a varied and balanced diet, it's important to stay hydrated and take any necessary prenatal supplements recommended by your healthcare provider. You can also find resources and support from vegan-friendly healthcare providers and online communities. Remember, every pregnancy is unique, and it's essential to prioritize your health and the health of your baby.

There have been studies on the long-term effects of veganism during pregnancy and breastfeeding. Some studies have suggested that vegan diets can be nutritionally adequate during pregnancy with proper planning and supplementation. However, it's important to note that veganism is not a one-size-fits-all approach, and individual needs may vary based on factors such as age, activity level, and health status.

It's recommended to work with a healthcare provider and a registered dietitian to ensure adequate nutrient intake during pregnancy and breastfeeding. Additionally, it's important to listen to your body and adjust your diet as needed to meet your individual needs.

CHAPTER 11

OVERCOMING COMMON CHALLENGES. DINING OUT, SOCIAL SITUATIONS, AND DEALING WITH CRAVINGS

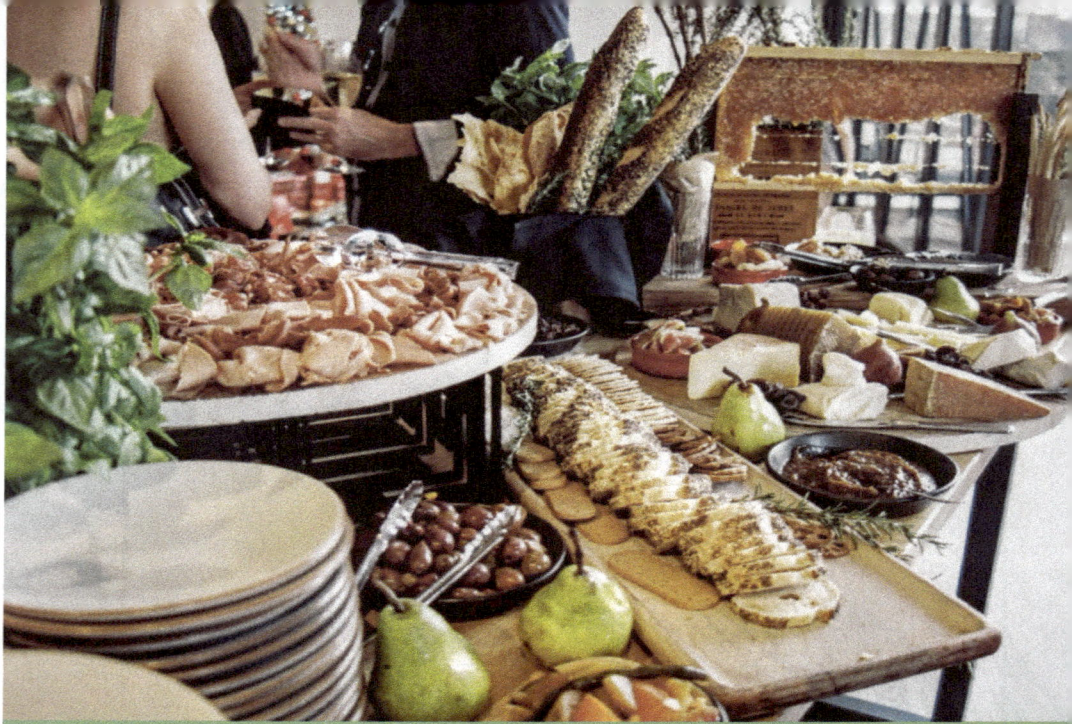

Now here is one of my favorite topics to talk about, given how I have experienced most of these struggles firsthand. As a vegan, dining out can present some challenges. One of the biggest challenges you may face is finding restaurants that offer vegan options or will accommodate your dietary needs. While many restaurants have vegan menus or can modify existing dishes to make them vegan-friendly, not all do.

Another issue with dining out is dealing with cross-contamination in the kitchen. This can happen when food preparation surfaces and utensils are shared between animal-based and plant-based dishes. To avoid this, it's important to let the restaurant know that you are vegan and ask about their food preparation practices.

You may also find that some restaurants simply don't understand what it means to be vegan and may offer you dishes that contain animal products, even if they think they are vegan. This can be frustrating, but it's important to remain clear and assertive about your dietary needs.

Finally, the lack of variety in vegan options at some restaurants can also be a challenge. While plant-based eating is becoming more popular, not all restaurants are keeping up with the trend. In these cases, you may need to get creative with ordering sides or modifying existing dishes to make them vegan-friendly.

Despite these challenges, with a bit of planning and communication, you can still enjoy dining out as a vegan. Don't be afraid to ask questions and advocate for yourself and remember that there are always delicious vegan options available if you know where to look!

In social situations, it can be helpful to bring your own vegan dish to share or offer to help with the meal planning to ensure there will be something for you to eat. You may also find it helpful to educate your friends and family about your reasons for going vegan and ask for their support.

Dealing with cravings can be another major challenge, but there are many delicious vegan alternatives that can help satisfy your cravings for meat, dairy, and other animal products. Yes, it was something to wrap my head around in the beginning but soon I found some vegan-friendly alternatives which I can always go to when craving something from my non-vegan days. For example, you can try plant-based burgers, vegan cheese, or dairy-free ice cream.

It's also important to remember why you chose to go vegan and focus on the positive impact it can have on your health, the environment, and animal welfare.

Surrounding yourself with supportive people and resources, such as online vegan communities or cookbooks, can also help you stay motivated and overcome common challenges. This is something that personally helped me whenever I felt overwhelmed.

Going vegan can elicit mixed reactions from friends and family, especially if they are not familiar with veganism or the reasons behind it. Some people may be supportive and curious, while others may be skeptical or even hostile. It's important to remember that everyone has their own journey and beliefs, and it's not your job to convince or force anyone to go vegan.

Instead, focus on being a positive example and sharing your knowledge and experiences in a respectful and non-judgmental manner. It may take time for others to come around, but the more you show them the benefits of veganism, the more likely they are to consider it for themselves. Ultimately, the decision to go vegan is a personal one, and it's up to everyone to make it for themselves based on their own values and beliefs.

CHAPTER 12:
"FAKE MEAT": WHY DO VEGANS EAT FAKE MEAT?

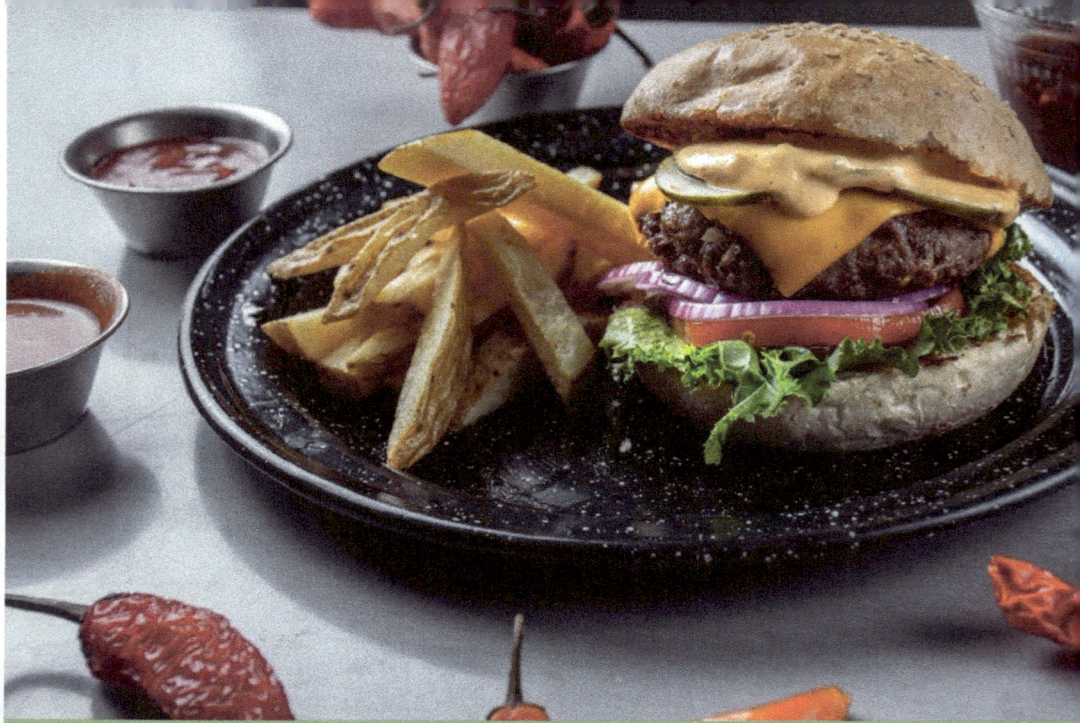

When on social media I see a lot of subtle attacks on Vegans from Non-Vegans. One attack is "Why do Vegans eat fake meat?"

Well, there's so much to say when someone asks this question so let's dive in!

Vegans may choose to eat fake meat for a variety of reasons. Some may enjoy the taste and texture of meat but want to avoid consuming animal products for ethical or environmental reasons. Others may be transitioning to a vegan diet and find that fake meats can help make the transition easier.

There are several reasons why people might choose to eat fake meat instead of conventional meat:

1. **Health concerns:** Some people may choose fake meat because it is typically lower in saturated fat and cholesterol than conventional meat, which can help reduce the risk of heart disease and other health problems.

2. **Environmental concerns:** Production of conventional meat has a significant environmental impact, including defor-estation, greenhouse gas emissions, and water pollution. By choosing plant-based meat, people can reduce their en-vironmental footprint.

3. **Animal welfare concerns:** Many people who choose fake meat do so because they are concerned about the treat-ment of animals in the meat industry.

4. **Taste preferences:** Some people simply prefer the taste and texture of plant-based meat over conventional meat.

Fake meat, also known as plant-based meat or meat alterna-tives, has become increasingly popular in recent years.

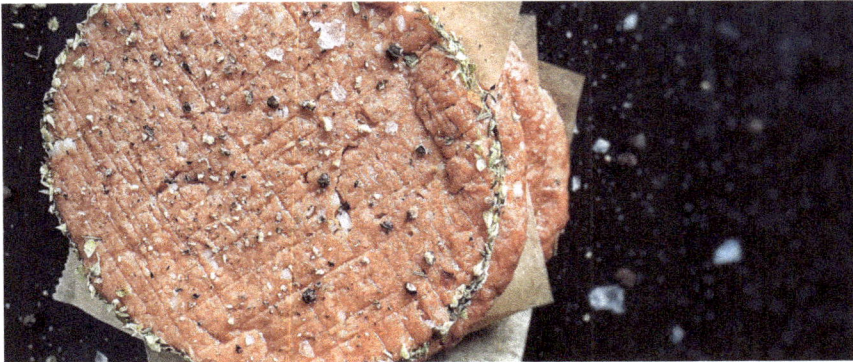

It is made from plant-based ingredients such as soy, wheat, and pea protein. They can be a good source of protein, iron, and other nutrients that are commonly found in meat. How-ever, it's important to note that not all fake meats are created equal in terms of nutrition. Some may be highly processed and contain large amounts of sodium and other additives.

The popularity of fake meat reflects a growing interest in sus-tainable, healthy, and ethical food choices. As technology improves, it is likely that plant-based meat will become even more realistic and appealing to consumers.

Overall, fake meats can be a convenient and satisfying food option for vegans, but they should be consumed in moderation as part of a balanced and varied diet. As with any food, it's important to read labels and choose products that are minimally processed and are nutrient dense.

CHAPTER 13:
VEGAN JUNK FOOD & HIGHLY PROCESSED FOODS

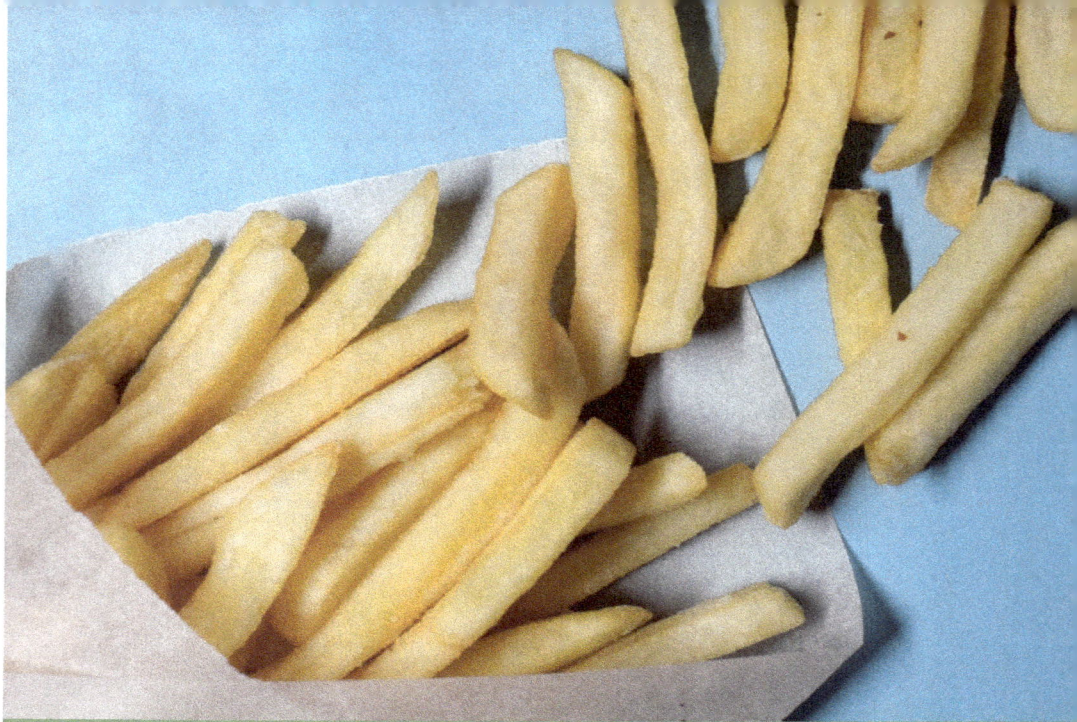

Ahhh this was so me in the beginning of my transition! I would grab some fries because it was convenient and delicious. Besides every restaurant and fast-food establishment serves fries!

A huge No No!

When transitioning to a vegan diet, it can be common to rely heavily on starchy foods such as French fries, pasta, and rice as they are often viewed as familiar and filling options. This diet I call the "Starch-atarian Diet". I'm very familiar with this diet. However, it's important to remember that while these foods can be a part of a healthy vegan diet, it's important to choose whole grain options and balance them with a variety of other nutrient-dense foods such as fruits, vegetables, legumes, nuts, and seeds.

Consuming a diverse range of plant-based foods ensures that you are getting all the necessary nutrients for optimal health, including protein, fiber, vitamins, and minerals. Additionally, incorporating physical activity into your daily routine can also help support a healthy transition to a vegan diet.

Then there are the highly processed foods like junk food. Yes, there is such a thing as highly processed vegan junk food. Just like with non-vegan junk food, processed vegan foods can be high in calories, sugar, salt, and unhealthy fats, and low in essential nutrients. Common examples of highly processed vegan junk food include:

- Vegan snack foods such as chips, pretzels, and crackers that are made with refined flour, added sugars, and artificial flavors and colors.
- Plant-based meat substitutes that are often made from isolated soy or other proteins, and contain added oils, salt, and flavorings to mimic the taste and texture of meat.
- Vegan desserts such as cookies, cakes, and ice-creams that are loaded with sugar and unhealthy fats.

While these foods may be vegan, they are not necessarily healthy or nutritious. Consuming too much highly processed vegan junk food can negatively impact your health, just like consuming too much non-vegan junk food can. It's important to prioritize whole, unprocessed plant-based foods in your diet to ensure that you are getting all the necessary nutrients for optimal health.

There are many vegan foods that are highly processed, regardless of whether they contain animal products or not. Some examples of highly processed vegan foods include vegan bacon, vegan cheese, vegan ice cream, and vegan frozen meals.

These types of foods often contain a high number of added sugars, unhealthy fats, and sodium, which can increase the risk of developing chronic diseases such as obesity, type 2 diabetes, and heart disease. In addition, many of these highly processed vegan foods may be low in essential nutrients such as fiber, vitamins, and minerals, which are important for maintaining good health.

Furthermore, many processed foods contain additives such as artificial colors, flavors, and preservatives, which may have harmful effects on our health. Some of these additives have been linked to allergic reactions, asthma, and even cancer.

It's important to note that not all vegan foods are highly processed, and many plant-based foods are naturally healthy and nutrient-dense. Examples of minimally processed vegan foods include fresh fruits and vegetables, whole grains, nuts, and seeds. When choosing vegan foods, it's important to read labels carefully and choose minimally processed options whenever possible to support optimal health.

Similarly, not all processed foods are unhealthy either, or some can be part of a balanced diet. Foods like canned vegetables, frozen fruits, and whole-grain bread are examples of processed foods that can be healthy options. However, it's important to read food labels carefully and choose minimally processed foods whenever possible. Overall, a diet that focuses on whole, unprocessed foods is the best way to support optimal health.

Highly processed vegan food may be recognizable by its packaging and ingredient list. Look for foods that have a long list of ingredients, especially if some of them are difficult to pronounce or recognize as whole foods. These may include additives and preservatives that are not natural, and they can also indicate that the food has been highly processed.

Another way to recognize highly processed vegan food is to check for added sugars and other sweeteners. Many processed vegan foods contain these additives to enhance flavor, which can lead to overconsumption of calories and contribute to health problems such as obesity and type 2 diabetes.

In addition to checking the ingredient list, you can look for highly processed vegan food by its appearance. Foods that are brightly colored or have an unnaturally uniform texture may have been highly processed, as natural vegan foods tend to vary in color, shape, and texture.

When you consume too many highly processed foods you miss out on key nutrients like fiber, vitamins, and minerals. Highly processed vegan foods may also be low in protein, which is essential for building and repairing tissues, and iron, which is important for carrying oxygen in the blood.

Fiber is an important nutrient that aids digestion, helps regulate blood sugar levels, and promotes feelings of fullness. Highly processed vegan foods may be low in fiber due to the removal of plant-based parts such as skins and seeds during processing.

Vitamins and minerals are also essential to overall health and wellness. For example, vitamin C is important for immune function and wound healing, while calcium is necessary for strong bones and teeth. Highly processed vegan foods may be lacking in these important nutrients due to the removal of natural sources during the manufacturing process.

It's important for vegans to be mindful of their nutrient intake and choose foods that will provide them with the necessary vitamins, minerals, and macronutrients for optimal health. This can be achieved by eating a variety of whole, plant-based foods and supplementing them with vitamins or fortified foods when necessary.

CHAPTER 14:
THE VEGAN KITCHEN: GROCERY LIST, COOKING TIPS AND RECIPES IDEAS

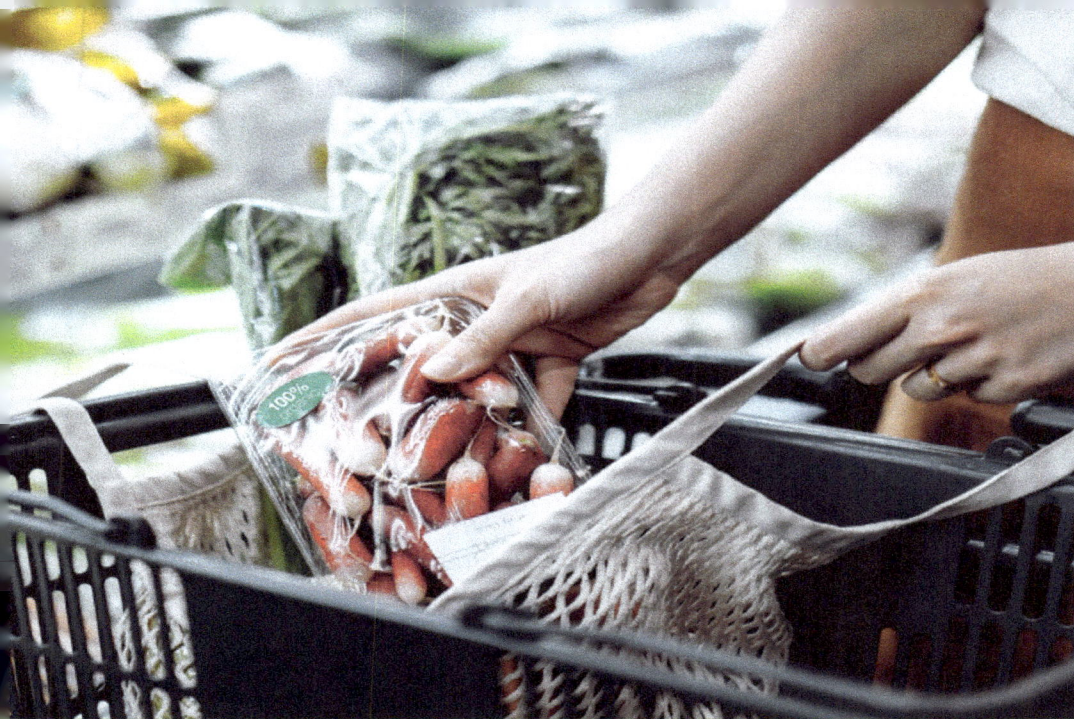

Grocery list
Your first all vegan grocery list:

(These are the basic ingredients some recipes will require further research)

Produce:

(Organic preferred)
- Spinach
- Kale
- Broccoli
- Carrots
- Bell peppers
- Onions
- Garlic
- Ginger
- Avocado

- Tomatoes
- Apples
- Bananas
- Berries
- Oranges
- Lemons
- Limes
-Cassava
-Sweet Potatoes
-Mushrooms

Protein:

- Tempeh
- Tofu
- Lentils
- Chickpeas

- Black beans
- Quinoa
-Seiten

Grains:

- Black rice
- Whole wheat pasta
-Chickpea Pasta

- Oats
- Bread
- Crackers

Nuts & Seeds:

- Almonds
- Cashews
- Walnuts
- Chia seeds

- Flax seeds
- Sunflower seeds
- Pumpkin seeds
- Nut butters

Dairy Alternatives:

(Choose one or two)
- Almond milk
- Coconut yogurt
- Cashew cheese

-Soy Milk
-Oat Milk
-Coconut Milk

Condiments & Spices:

- Olive oil
- Balsamic vinegar
- Soy sauce
- Hot sauce
- Mustard

- Ketchup
- Herbs (basil, thyme, rosemary)
- Spices (cumin, chili powder, paprika)

Ingredients for Baking: (As needed)

-Non-dairy milk (such as almond, soy, or oat milk)

- Vegan butter or margarine

- Coconut oil or vegetable oil

- Applesauce or mashed bananas (as a replacement for eggs in some recipes)

- Agave nectar, maple syrup, or other plant-based sweeteners

- Aquafaba (liquid from a can of chickpeas that can be whipped into a meringue-like consistency)

- Vegan chocolate chips or chunks

- Nutritional yeast (for adding a cheesy flavor to dishes)

- Silken tofu (can be blended into creamy desserts like cheesecake)

- Vegan cream cheese or sour cream (for frosting and other baked goods)

-All-purpose flour

-Whole wheat flour

-Spelt flour

-Oat flour

-Coconut flour.

Frozen Foods:

- Organic Frozen fruits and vegetables (for smoothies or stir-fry)

This list should provide a good foundation for a 30-day vegan diet plan. However, please note that individual dietary needs may vary and it's important to consult a healthcare professional before making any significant changes to your diet.

Disclaimer: These recipes may contain nuts or nut-based ingredients. Please be aware of this if you have a nut allergy and use caution when preparing or consuming these dishes.

1: Vegan Waffles

Ingredients:

- 1 tbsp ground flaxseed
- 3 tbsp water
- 1 1/2 cups all-purpose flour
- 2 tbsp sugar
- 1 tbsp baking powder
- 1/4 tsp salt
- 1 1/4 cups plant-based milk
- 1/3 cup vegetable oil
- 1 tsp vanilla extract

Instructions:

1. In a small bowl, whisk together the flaxseed and water. Let it sit for a few minutes to thicken.

2. In a separate bowl, mix the flour, sugar, baking powder, and salt.

3. Add the plant-based milk, vegetable oil, and vanilla extract to the bowl with the flaxseed mixture and stir to combine.

4. Pour the wet ingredients into the dry ingredients and mix until just combined (it's okay if there are a few lumps).

5. Heat up your waffle iron and spray it with cooking spray.

6. Cook the waffles according to the instructions on your waffle iron, until they're golden brown and crispy.

7. Serve with your desired toppings.

Vegan Bacon Recipes:

2: Tempeh Bacon

Ingredients:

- 8 oz tempeh
- 1/4 cup soy sauce
- 2 tbsp liquid smoke
- 2 tbsp maple syrup or agave nectar
- 1 tsp smoked paprika

- Freshly ground black pepper

- Vegetable oil for frying

Instructions:

1. Slice the tempeh into thin pieces.

2. In a shallow dish, whisk together the soy sauce, liquid smoke, maple syrup, smoked paprika, and black pepper.

3. Add the tempeh slices to the marinade and let them sit for at least 30 minutes.

4. Heat some vegetable oil in a non-stick skillet over medium-high heat.

5. Add the tempeh slices to the skillet and fry for 2-3 minutes per side, or until crispy and browned.

6. Serve immediately.

3: Coconut Bacon

Ingredients:

- 2 cups unsweetened coconut flakes

- 2 tbsp soy sauce

- 1 tbsp liquid smoke

- 1 tbsp maple syrup

- 1 tsp smoked paprika

Instructions:

1. Preheat your oven to 325°F (160°C).

2. In a large bowl, mix the coconut flakes, soy sauce, liquid smoke, maple syrup, and smoked paprika.

3. Spread the mixture out in a single layer on a baking sheet lined with parchment paper.

4. Bake for 20-25 minutes, stirring every 5 minutes, until the coconut is crispy and browned.

5. Serve immediately or store in an airtight container for up to a week.

4: Mushroom Bacon

Ingredients:

- 8 oz mushrooms (cremini or shiitake)
- 1/4 cup soy sauce
- 2 tbsp apple cider vinegar
- 2 tsp liquid smoke
- 1 tsp garlic powder
- Vegetable oil for frying

Instructions:

1. Slice the mushrooms into thin pieces.

2. In a shallow dish, whisk together the soy sauce, apple cider vinegar, liquid smoke, and garlic powder.

3. Add the mushroom slices to the marinade and let them sit for at least 30 minutes.

4. Heat some vegetable oil in a non-stick skillet over medium-high heat.

5. Add the mushroom slices to the skillet and fry for 2-3 minutes per side, or until crispy and browned.

6. Serve immediately.

5: Vegan Bacon

Ingredients:

- 1 block firm tofu
- 3 tbsp soy sauce
- 1 tbsp maple syrup
- 1/2 tsp liquid smoke
- 1/2 tsp garlic powder
- 1/4 tsp smoked paprika
- Salt and pepper to taste

Instructions:

1. Drain the tofu and slice it into thin strips.

2. In a shallow dish, whisk together the soy sauce, maple syrup, liquid smoke, garlic powder, smoked paprika, salt, and pepper.

3. Add the tofu slices to the marinade and let them sit for at least 30 minutes.

4. Heat some vegetable oil in a non-stick skillet over medium-high heat.

5. Add the tofu slices to the skillet and fry for 2-3 minutes per side, or until crispy and browned.

6. Serve immediately.

6: Blueberry Pancakes

Ingredients:

- 1 cup flour
- 2 tsp baking powder
- 1 tbsp sugar
- 1/4 tsp salt
- 1 cup almond milk
- 2 tbsp melted coconut oil
- 1 tsp vanilla extract
- 1 cup blueberries

Instructions:

1. In a medium bowl, whisk together the flour, baking powder, sugar, and salt.

2. In a separate bowl, whisk together the almond milk, coconut oil, and vanilla extract.

3. Add the wet ingredients to the dry ingredients and stir until just combined.

4. Gently fold in the blueberries.

5. Heat a non-stick skillet over medium heat and lightly grease with oil or non-stick spray.

6. Pour about 1/4 cup batter onto the skillet for each pancake.

7. Cook until bubbles form on the surface of the pancake, then flip and cook for an additional minute or two.

8. Serve hot with syrup and additional blueberries if desired.

7: Chocolate Peanut Butter Smoothie Bowl

Ingredients:

- 1 frozen banana
- 1 cup almond milk
- 1 tbsp cocoa powder
- 1 tbsp peanut butter
- 1 tbsp maple syrup
- Toppings such as sliced banana, chopped nuts, or shredded coconut

Instructions:

1. Blend the frozen banana, almond milk, cocoa powder, peanut butter, and maple syrup in a blender until smooth.

2. Pour the smoothie into a bowl and top with desired toppings.

Recipe 7: Veggie Omelet

Ingredients:

- 1/2 cup chickpea flour
- 1/2 cup water
- Salt and pepper to taste
- 1/4 cup diced bell pepper
- 1/4 cup diced onion
- 1/4 cup diced mushroom
- 1 tbsp nutritional yeast
- Fresh herbs such as parsley or basil

Instructions:

1. In a medium bowl, whisk together the chickpea flour, water, salt, and pepper until smooth.

2. Stir in the bell pepper, onion, mushroom, and nutritional yeast.

3. Heat a non-stick skillet over medium heat and lightly grease with oil or non-stick spray.

4. Pour the mixture onto the skillet and cook for about 3-4 minutes on each side, or until golden brown.

5. Top with fresh herbs before serving.

8: Strawberry Overnight Oats

Ingredients:

- 1/2 cup rolled oats
- 1/2 cup almond milk
- 1/2 cup diced strawberries
- 1 tbsp chia seeds
- 1 tbsp maple syrup
- Dash of vanilla extract

Instructions:

1. In a jar or bowl, mix the oats, almond milk, strawberries, chia seeds, maple syrup, and vanilla extract.

2. Cover and refrigerate overnight.

3. In the morning, stir the mixture and add additional almond milk if needed.

4. Serve cold with additional strawberries if desired.

9: Tofu Scramble

Ingredients:

- 1 block firm tofu
- 1 tbsp olive oil
- 1/4 cup diced onion
- 1/4 cup diced bell pepper
- 1/4 cup diced mushroom
- 1 tsp turmeric
- Salt and pepper to taste

Instructions:

1. Drain the tofu and crumble it into a bowl.

2. Heat the olive oil in a non-stick skillet over medium heat.

3. Add the onion, bell pepper, and mushroom and cook until softened.

4. Add the crumbled tofu, turmeric, salt, and pepper and stir to combine.

5. Cook for about 5-7 minutes, or until heated through.

6. Serve hot with toast or hash browns.

10: Cinnamon French Toast

Ingredients:

- 4 slices bread (preferably day-old)
- 1 cup almond milk
- 1 tbsp cornstarch
- 1 tsp vanilla extract
- 1/2 tsp cinnamon
- 1 tbsp maple syrup
- Vegan butter for frying

Instructions:

1. In a shallow dish, whisk together the almond milk, cornstarch, vanilla extract, cinnamon, and maple syrup until smooth.

2. Heat a non-stick skillet over medium heat and melt some vegan butter.

3. Dip each slice of bread into the almond milk mixture, making sure to coat both sides.

4. Fry the bread for about 2-3 minutes on each side, or until golden brown.

5. Serve hot with additional maple syrup if desired.

11: Vegan Breakfast Burrito

Ingredients:

- 1/2 cup black beans
- 1/4 cup diced tomato
- 1/4 cup diced onion
- 1/4 cup diced bell pepper
- 1/2 tsp chili powder
- Salt and pepper to taste
- 1 large flour tortilla
- Salsa and avocado for serving

Instructions:

1. Heat a non-stick skillet over medium heat.

2. Add the black beans, tomato, onion, bell pepper, chili powder, salt, and pepper and cook until heated through.

3. Warm the flour tortilla in the microwave or on the stove.

4. Spoon the bean mixture onto the tortilla and top with salsa and avocado.

5. Roll up the burrito and serve hot.

12: Vegan BLT w/Cheese Sandwich

Ingredients:

- 1 English muffin
- 1 slice of firm tofu
- Vegan cheese slice

- Vegan bacon (from recipe above)
- Salt and pepper to taste

- Lettuce
-Slice tomato

Instructions:

1. Toast the English muffin.

2. Slice the tofu into rounds and fry in a non-stick skillet until golden brown.

3. Top one half of the English muffin with the vegan cheese, lettuce and tomato.

4. Top the other half of the English muffin with tofu and vegan bacon.

5. Season with salt and pepper to taste.

6. Put the two halves together to make the sandwich and serve hot.

13: Banana Nut Bread

Ingredients:

- 1 cup flour
- 1 tsp baking soda
- 1/4 tsp salt
- 3 ripe bananas, mashed
- 1/3 cup melted coconut oil

- 1/2 cup brown sugar
- 1 tbsp ground flaxseed mixed with3
- 3 tbsp water
- 1/2 cup chopped walnuts

Instructions:

1. Preheat your oven to 350°F (175°C) and grease a loaf pan.

2. In a medium bowl, whisk together the flour, baking soda, and salt.

3. In a separate large bowl, mix the mashed bananas, melted coconut oil, and brown sugar.

4. Add the dry ingredients into the wet mixture and stir until well combined.

5. In a small bowl, mix the flaxseed and water to make a "flax egg". Stir this into the batter.

6. Fold in the chopped walnuts.

7. Pour the batter into the prepared loaf pan.

8. Bake for 50-60 minutes, or until a toothpick inserted into the center comes out clean.

9. Allow the bread to cool in the pan for a few minutes before removing and slicing. Enjoy warm or at room temperature!

14: Vegan Breakfast Burrito

Ingredients:

- 1 large tortilla wrap
- 1/4 cup black beans
- 1/4 cup diced tomato
- 1 small avocado, sliced
- 2 tbsp salsa
- salt and pepper to taste

Instructions:

1. Warm up the tortilla wrap in the microwave or in a skillet.

2. Add the black beans, diced tomato, sliced avocado, and salsa on top of the tortilla.

3. Season with salt and pepper to taste.

4. Fold the bottom of the tortilla up over the filling, then fold in the sides and roll up tightly.

5. Serve hot and enjoy!

15: Blueberry Oatmeal

Ingredients:

- 1 cup rolled oats
- 2 cups water
- 1/4 cup blueberries
- 2 tbsp maple syrup
- 1 tbsp chia seeds
- 1 tsp vanilla extract
- pinch of salt

Instructions:

1. In a small saucepan, bring the water to a boil.

2. Add the rolled oats and salt, reduce heat to low, and simmer for 10-12 minutes, stirring occasionally.

3. Stir in the blueberries, maple syrup, chia seeds, and vanilla extract until well combined.

4. Cook for an additional 2-3 minutes until the oatmeal is thick and creamy.

5. Serve hot and enjoy!

16: Vegan Banana Pancakes

Ingredients:

- 1 ripe banana, mashed
- 1/2 cup flour
- 1/2 cup almond milk
- 1 tsp baking powder
- 1/2 tsp cinnamon
- 1/4 tsp salt

Instructions:

1. In a mixing bowl, combine the mashed banana, flour, almond milk, baking powder, cinnamon, and salt.

2. Mix until well combined and smooth.

3. Heat a non-stick skillet over medium heat.

4. Drop 1/4 cup of batter onto the skillet for each pancake.

5. Cook for 2-3 minutes until bubbles appear on the surface.

6. Flip the pancake and cook for an additional 1-2 minutes until golden brown.

7. Repeat with the remaining batter.

8. Serve hot with your favorite toppings and enjoy!

17: Vegan Chickun and Waffles

Ingredients:

- 1 cup vegan chicken pieces
- 1 cup all-purpose flour
- 1 tablespoon sugar
- 2 teaspoons baking powder
- 1/2 teaspoon salt
- 1 cup unsweetened almond milk
- 1/4 cup coconut oil, melted
- 1 teaspoon vanilla extract
- Maple syrup, for serving

Instructions:

1. In a large mixing bowl, whisk together the flour, sugar, baking powder, and salt.

2. Add the almond milk, melted coconut oil, and vanilla extract to the dry ingredients. Mix until just combined.

3. Preheat a non-stick waffle maker and brush with coconut oil.

4. Cook the vegan chicken pieces in a frying pan over medium-high heat until crispy and browned on all sides.

5. Pour the waffle batter onto the preheated waffle maker and cook until golden brown. Repeat until all the batter is used up.

6. To serve, place a waffle on a plate and top with the crispy vegan chicken. Drizzle with maple syrup and any other desired toppings.

18: Vegan Smoothie Bowl

Ingredients:

- 1 frozen banana
- 1/2 cup frozen mixed berries
- 1/2 cup almond milk
- 1 tbsp chia seeds
- 1/4 cup granola
- 1 tbsp peanut butter

Instructions:

1. In a blender, combine the frozen banana, frozen mixed berries, almond milk, and chia seeds.

2. Blend until smooth and creamy.

3. Pour the smoothie into a bowl and top with granola and peanut butter.

4. Serve immediately and enjoy!

19: Vegan Breakfast Cookies

Ingredients:

- 1 cup rolled oats
- 1/2 cup flour

- 1/2 cup almond butter
- 1/4 cup maple syrup
- 1/4 cup almond milk
- 1 tsp baking powder

- 1/2 tsp cinnamon
- pinch of salt
- 1/4 cup dried cranberries

Instructions:

1. Preheat your oven to 350°F (175°C) and line a baking sheet with parchment paper.

2. In a mixing bowl, combine the rolled oats, flour, almond butter, maple syrup, almond milk, baking powder, cinnamon, and salt.

3. Stir until well combined and smooth.

4. Fold in the dried cranberries.

5. Scoop the batter onto the baking sheet using a cookie scoop or spoon.

6. Flatten each cookie slightly with a fork.

7. Bake for 12-15 minutes until golden brown.

8. Allow the cookies to cool on the baking sheet for a few minutes before transferring to a wire rack.

9. Serve warm or at room temperature and enjoy!

20: Vegan Grits and Chickpea Scrambled

Ingredients:

- 1 cup yellow grits
- 4 cups water
- 1 teaspoon salt
- 1 tablespoon olive oil
- 1 onion, chopped
- 2 cloves garlic, minced
- 1 red bell pepper, chopped
- 1 can chickpeas, drained and rinsed

- 1/2 teaspoon cumin
- 1/2 teaspoon chili powder
- Salt and black pepper to taste

Instructions:

For the vegan grits:

1. In a large saucepan, bring 4 cups of water to a boil.

2. Add 1 teaspoon salt and slowly stir in 1 cup of yellow grits.

3. Reduce heat to low and cover, stirring occasionally until the grits are creamy and tender, about 15-20 minutes.

For the vegan chickpea scrambled:

1. Heat olive oil in a large non-stick skillet over medium-high heat.

2. Sauté onions and garlic until they are soft and translucent, about 3-5 minutes.

3. Add red bell pepper and cook until tender, another 3-5 minutes.

4. Stir in chickpeas, cumin, chili powder, salt, and black pepper to the skillet and cook until heated through, about 5-8 minutes.

5. Serve hot vegan chickpea scrambled over a bed of creamy vegan grits.

21: Vegan Avocado Toast

Ingredients:

- 1 slice of bread
- 1/2 avocado, mashed
- squeeze of fresh lemon juice
- salt and pepper to taste
- optional toppings: cherry tomatoes, red onion, microgreens

Instructions:

1. Toast your bread to your desired level of crispiness.

2. In a small bowl, mash the avocado with a fork.

3. Squeeze in some fresh lemon juice and season with salt and pepper to taste.

4. Spread the mashed avocado on top of the toast.

5. Add any optional toppings you prefer.

6. Serve immediately and enjoy!

22: Vegan Banana Bread Oatmeal

Ingredients:

- 1 cup rolled oats
- 2 cups water
- 1 ripe banana, mashed
- 2 tbsp maple syrup
- 1 tsp vanilla extract
- pinch of salt
- 1/4 cup chopped walnuts

Instructions:

1. In a small saucepan, bring the water to a boil.

2. Add the rolled oats and salt, reduce heat to low, and simmer for 10-12 minutes, stirring occasionally.

3. Stir in the mashed banana, maple syrup, and vanilla extract until well combined.

4. Cook for an additional 2-3 minutes until the oatmeal is thick and creamy.

5. Fold in the chopped walnuts.

6. Serve hot and enjoy!

Recipe 23: Vegan Breakfast Tacos

Ingredients:

- 6 small corn tortillas
- 1 can of black beans, drained and rinsed
- 1/2 tsp cumin
- 1/4 tsp paprika
- 1/4 tsp garlic powder
- salt and pepper, to taste
- 1/2 avocado, sliced
- salsa, to taste
- fresh cilantro, chopped

Instructions:

1. In a large skillet over medium heat, add the black beans and spices. Cook for 5-7 minutes until heated through and well-seasoned.

2. Warm the corn tortillas on a separate skillet or in the microwave.

3. Assemble the tacos by layering the seasoned black beans, sliced avocado, salsa, and fresh cilantro on top of each warmed tortilla.

4. Serve immediately and enjoy your delicious Vegan Breakfast Tacos!

24: Vegan Pancakes

Ingredients:

- 1 tbsp ground flaxseed

- 3 tbsp water

- 1 cup all-purpose flour

- 2 tbsp sugar

- 2 tsp baking powder

- 1/4 tsp salt

- 1 cup plant-based milk

- 2 tbsp vegetable oil

- 1 tsp vanilla extract

- Optional toppings: sliced bananas, fresh blueberries, chocolate chips

Instructions:

1. In a small bowl, whisk together the flaxseed and water. Let it sit for a few minutes to thicken.

2. In a separate bowl, mix the flour, sugar, baking powder, and salt.

3. Add the plant-based milk, vegetable oil, and vanilla extract to the bowl with the flaxseed mixture and stir to combine.

4. Pour the wet ingredients into the dry ingredients and mix until just combined (it's okay if there are a few lumps).

5. Heat a non-stick skillet over medium heat. Add a ladleful of batter and cook until bubbles appear on the surface. Flip and cook for another minute or until golden brown.

6. Serve with your desired toppings.

25: Apple Oat Pancakes

Ingredients:

- 1 cup rolled oats.
- 1/2 teaspoon baking powder
- 2 tablespoons maple syrup
- 1/2 teaspoon ground cinnamon
- 1 apple (peeled, cored and finely diced)
- 1/4 cup almond milk

Instructions:

1. Combine all ingredients in a large bowl and mix until everything is well incorporated.

2. Heat a non-stick skillet over medium heat.

3. scoop batter onto skillet and cook until lightly browned, flipping halfway.

4. Serve pancakes with your favorite toppings.

26: Vegan Seasoned Hash Browns

Ingredients:

- 4 medium-sized potatoes, peeled and grated
- 1/2 cup all-purpose flour
- 1/4 cup nutritional yeast
- 1/2 teaspoon garlic powder
- 1/2 teaspoon onion powder
- 1/2 teaspoon smoked paprika
- Salt and black pepper to taste
- 2 tablespoons avocado oil

Instructions:

1. In a large bowl, mix grated potatoes, all-purpose flour, nutritional yeast, garlic powder, onion powder, smoked paprika, salt, and black pepper until well combined.

2. Heat avocado oil in a large non-stick skillet over medium-high heat.

3. Form potato mixture into flat patties and gently place them in the hot skillet.

4. Cook each side until golden brown and crispy, about 4-5 minutes per side.

5. Serve hot vegan seasoned hash browns as a side dish or breakfast.

27: Coconut Yogurt Parfait

Ingredients:

- 2/3 cup coconut yogurt
- 1/4 cup granola

- 1/4 cup diced mango.

Instructions:

1. Layer yogurt

2. Granola and mango in a glass or bowl.

Recipe 28: Overnight Oats

Ingredients:

- 1/2 cup rolled oats.
- 1/2 cup almond milk
- 1/2 teaspoon ground cinnamon

- 1/4 cup chopped apples.
- 2 tablespoons honey

Instructions:

1. Combine all ingredients in a mason jar or bowl and stir to combine.

2. Cover and refrigerate overnight. Enjoy in the morning!

29: Chickpea Flour Omelet

Ingredients:

- 1 cup chickpea flour
- 1 cup water
- 1 tbsp olive oil

- 1/4 tsp salt
- 1/4 tsp turmeric
- 1/4 tsp black pepper

- 1/2 cup sautéed vegetables (mushrooms, onions, bell peppers, etc.)

- Avocado, salsa, or vegan cheese for topping

Instructions:

1. In a bowl, whisk together the chickpea flour, water, olive oil, salt, turmeric, and black pepper until smooth.

2. Heat a nonstick skillet over medium heat and add a little oil. Pour half of the batter into the pan and spread it out evenly.

3. Cook for 2-3 minutes until the edges start to lift and the bottom is set.

4. Add your sautéed vegetables on one side of the omelet and use a spatula to fold the other side over to cover them.

5. Slide the omelet onto a plate and top with avocado, salsa, or vegan cheese.

30: Vegan Biscuits

Ingredients:

- 2 cups all-purpose flour

- 1 tbsp baking powder

- 1 tsp salt

- 1/4 cup vegan butter, chilled and cubed

- 3/4 cup non-dairy milk (such as almond or soy milk)

- 1 tbsp apple cider vinegar

Instructions:

1. Preheat the oven to 425°F (218°C) and line a baking sheet with parchment paper.

2. In a large mixing bowl, whisk together the flour, baking powder, and salt.

3. Add the chilled vegan butter and use a pastry cutter or

your hands to mix it in until the mixture resembles coarse crumbs.

4. In a separate bowl, whisk together the non-dairy milk and apple cider vinegar. Add this mixture to the flour mixture and stir until just combined. Do not over-mix.

5. Turn the dough out onto a floured surface and knead gently for 1-2 minutes until it comes together.

6. Use your hands to flatten the dough to about 1 inch thick. Use a biscuit cutter or a glass to cut out biscuits and place them on the prepared baking sheet.

7. Bake for 12-15 minutes until golden brown.

8. Serve warm and enjoy!

Tip: For extra deliciousness, brush the tops of the biscuits with melted vegan butter before baking.

Disclaimer: These recipes may contain nuts or nut-based ingredients. Please be aware of this if you have a nut allergy and use caution when preparing or consuming these dishes.

30 Vegan Snack Ideas

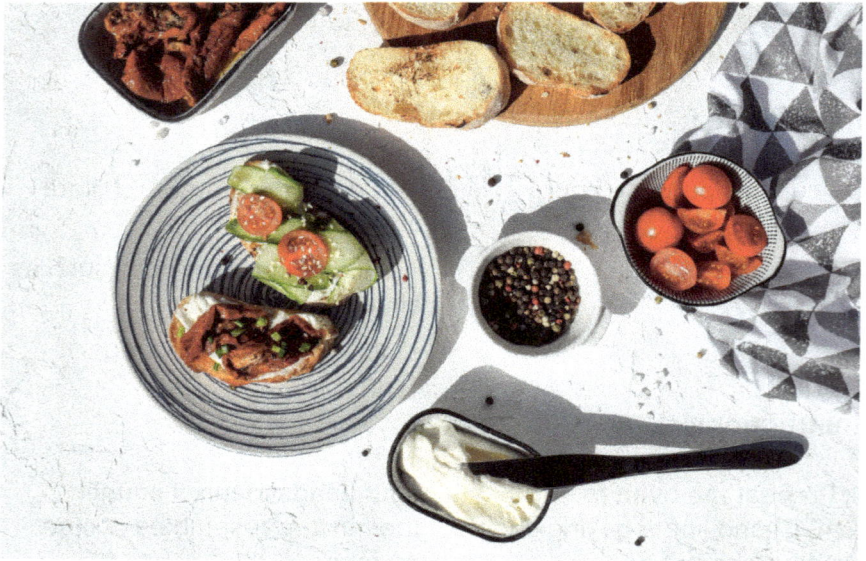

1. Hummus and Pita Chips

Dip pita chips in homemade or store-bought hummus or Homemade.

2. Fruit Salad

Mix chopped fruit, such as strawberries, kiwi, pineapple, and grapes, for a refreshing snack.

3. Almond Butter Energy Balls

Mix almond butter, oats, honey or maple syrup, and chocolate chips, then roll into bite-sized balls.

4. Roasted Chickpeas

Toss canned chickpeas with cumin and garlic powder, then bake at 400°F for 20-25 minutes until crispy.

5. Veggie Smoothie

Blend spinach, kale, banana, and almond milk for a nutritious, filling snack.

6. Avocado Toast

Spread mashed avocado on whole grain bread or a rice cake, then sprinkle with salt and pepper.

7. Vegan Trail Mix

Mix nuts, seeds, dried fruit, and dark chocolate for a portable snack.

8. Baked Sweet Potato Fries

Slice sweet potatoes into fries, toss with olive oil and paprika, then place in Air Fryer or bake at 400°F for 20-25 minutes until crispy.

9. Guacamole and Veggie Chips

Mash avocado with lime juice, garlic, and salt, then serve with veggie chips.

10. Carrot and Apple Slices with Nut Butter

Dip sliced carrots and apples into your favorite nut butter.

11. Vegetable Soup

Heat up a vegetable-based soup for a warming snack.

12. Energy bars

Choose vegan energy bars made with whole food ingredients.

13. Edamame

Steam edamame pods and sprinkle light with sea salt.

14. Apple Slices with cinnamon

Sprinkle cinnamon on apple slices for a sweet and spicy snack.

15. Vegan cheese and crackers

Pair vegan cheese with whole grain crackers for a savory snack.

16. Raw Veggies and Dip

Serve raw veggies like carrot sticks and cucumber with vegan dip.

17. Pumpkin seeds

Roast pumpkin seeds for a crunchy snack.

18. Vegan Smoothie Bowl

Blend frozen fruit, almond milk, and protein powder, then top with granola and fresh fruit.

19. Baked Kale Chips

Toss kale with olive oil and salt, then bake at 350°F for 10-15 minutes until crispy.

20. Oatmeal with fruit and nuts

Mix oats with almond milk, chia seeds, and sliced fruit, then top with nuts for a filling snack.

21. Celery sticks with peanut butter

Spread peanut butter on celery sticks.

22. Roasted sweet potato chips

Slice a sweet potato thinly, toss with olive oil and salt, then roast in the oven at 400°F for 15-20 minutes until crispy.

23. Chia seed pudding

Mix chia seeds with almond milk, vanilla extract, and a sweetener of your choice (ex. honey, maple syrup), then refrigerate overnight.

24. Baked apple chips

Slice apples thinly, sprinkle with cinnamon, and bake in the oven at 200°F for 2-3 hours until crispy.

25. Kale and White Bean Dip

Blend blanched kale, white beans, garlic, lemon juice, and olive oil in a food processor until smooth.

26. Zucchini chips

Slice zucchini thinly, toss with olive oil and salt, then bake in the oven at 350°F for 10-15 minutes until crispy.

27. Cucumber and Tomato Salad

Slice cucumbers and tomatoes, then toss with olive oil, lemon juice, salt, and pepper.

28. Steamed Artichoke

Steam a whole artichoke until tender, then dip the leaves in lemon-garlic vegan butter.

29. Hummus and Veggie Sticks

Dip carrot sticks, cucumber slices, and bell pepper strips in hummus.

30. Energy balls

Blend dates, almond butter, rolled oats, and any mix-ins you like (ex. shredded coconut, cocoa powder, chopped nuts) in a food processor, then roll into balls.

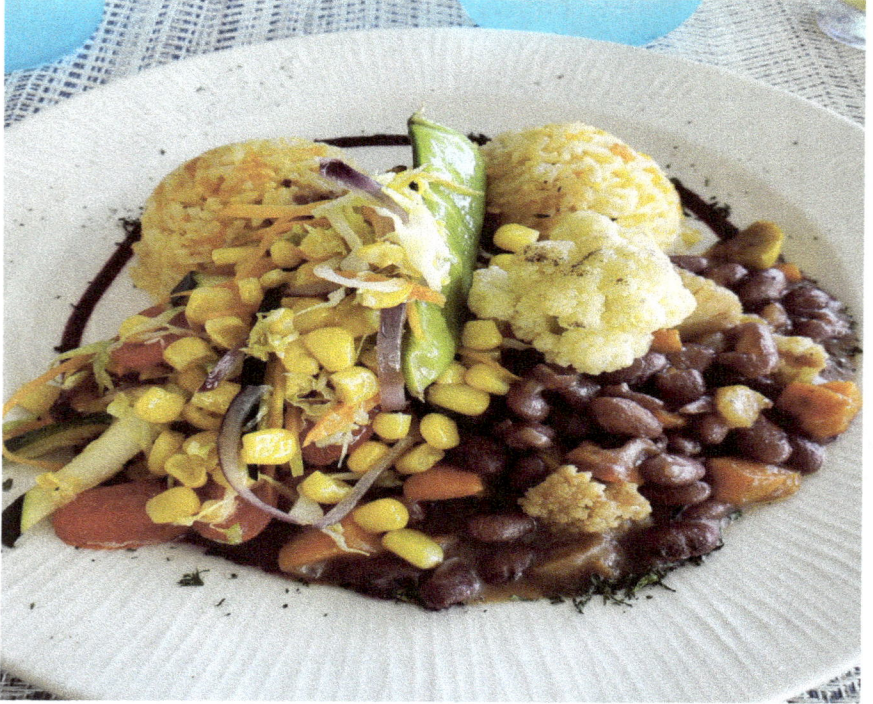

1. Vegan Chili with Cornbread

Ingredients:

- 2 tbsp olive oil

- 1 onion, diced

- 3 cloves garlic, minced

- 1 red bell pepper, diced

- 1 green bell pepper, diced

- 1 jalapeño pepper, seeded and diced

- 1 can kidney beans, drained and rinsed

- 1 can black beans, drained and rinsed

- 1 can diced tomatoes

- 1 tbsp chili powder

- 1 tsp ground cumin

- Salt and pepper to taste

- Cornbread mix (prepared according to package instructions)

Instructions:

1. Preheat oven to 350°F.

2. In a large pot, heat olive oil over medium heat. Add onion, garlic, and peppers and cook until tender.

3. Add beans, tomatoes, chili powder, cumin, salt, and pepper. Stir well.

4. Reduce heat and simmer for 20 minutes.

5. Pour the chili into an 8-inch square baking dish.

6. Prepare the cornbread mix according to the package instructions, then pour the batter on top of the chili.

7. Bake for 30 minutes or until the cornbread is golden brown.

2. Tofu Stir-Fry with Veggies and Rice

Ingredients:

- 1 block extra firm tofu, drained and cut into cubes

- 1 tbsp sesame oil

- 2 cloves garlic, minced

- 1 tbsp ginger, peeled and minced

- 1 red bell pepper, sliced into thin strips

- 1 yellow bell pepper, sliced into thin strips

- 1 green bell pepper, sliced into thin strips

- 2 cups snow peas

- 1 tbsp soy sauce

- 1 tbsp hoisin sauce

- 1 tbsp rice vinegar

- Salt and pepper to taste

- Cooked rice

Instructions:

1. Heat sesame oil in a large skillet over medium-high heat.

2. Add tofu and sauté until lightly browned, about 5 minutes.

3. Add garlic and ginger and cook for another 2 minutes.

4. Add bell peppers and snow peas, and sauté for 5-7 minutes.

5. In a small bowl, whisk together soy sauce, hoisin sauce, and rice vinegar. Pour the

mixture over the vegetables and toss to coat.

6. Serve hot over cooked rice.

3. Vegan Roasted Vegetable Lasagna

Ingredients:

- 1 eggplant, sliced into 1/4" rounds

- 1 zucchini, sliced into 1/4" rounds

- 1 yellow squash, sliced into 1/4" rounds

- 1 red onion, sliced into thin rounds

- 2 tbsp olive oil

- Salt and pepper to taste

- 8 lasagna noodles

- 2 cups marinara sauce

- 1 cup vegan ricotta cheese

- 1/2 cup vegan mozzarella cheese, shredded

- Fresh basil, chopped (optional)

Instructions:

1. Preheat oven to 375°F.

2. Arrange the eggplant, zucchini, yellow squash, and red onion on a baking sheet. Drizzle with olive oil and sprinkle with salt and pepper. Bake for 20-25 minutes, or until vegetables are tender and lightly browned.

3. Cook lasagna noodles according to package instructions.

4. Spread a thin layer of marinara sauce on the bottom of a 9-inch square baking dish.

5. Layer lasagna noodles on top of sauce.

6. Spread a layer of roasted vegetables on top of the noodles, then add a layer of vegan ricotta cheese.

7. Repeat until all ingredients are used up.

8. Sprinkle vegan mozzarella cheese on top.

9. Bake for 30-35 minutes, or until lasagna is hot and bubbly.

10. Let cool for a few minutes, then sprinkle with chopped fresh basil (optional) before serving.

4. Vegan Lentil Soup

Ingredients:

- 1 tbsp olive oil
- 1 onion, diced
- 3 cloves garlic, minced
- 2 carrots, diced
- 2 celery stalks, diced
- 1 cup brown lentils
- 6 cups vegetable broth
- 1 bay leaf
- Salt and pepper to taste
- Fresh parsley, chopped (optional)

Instructions:

1. Heat olive oil in a large pot over medium heat.

2. Add onion and garlic and cook until onion is translucent.

3. Add carrots and celery and cook for another 5-7 minutes.

4. Add lentils, vegetable broth, and bay leaf. Bring to a boil, then reduce heat and simmer for 30-40 minutes, or until lentils are tender.

5. Discard Bay leaf and season with salt and pepper to taste.

6. Allow soup to cool for a few minutes, then blend until smooth using an immersion blender or transfer in batches to a blender.

7. Return soup to pot and reheat if necessary. Serve hot, garnished with chopped fresh parsley if desired.

5. Vegan BBQ jackfruit tacos:

Ingredients:

- 1 can of jackfruit in water or brine
- 1/2 cup BBQ sauce
- Salt and pepper to taste
- Corn tortillas
- Optional toppings: diced avocado, chopped cilantro, sliced jalapeños

Instructions:

1. Drain jackfruit and rinse thoroughly.

2. Add jackfruit to a skillet over medium heat and cook until slightly browned, about 5 minutes.

3. Add BBQ sauce and stir to coat jackfruit.

4. Reduce heat to low and simmer for 10-15 minutes, or until jackfruit has absorbed the BBQ sauce.

5. Season with salt and pepper to taste.

6. Warm the corn tortillas and assemble the tacos with the jackfruit mixture and desired toppings. Serve and enjoy!

6. Vegan spaghetti carbonara with cashew cream sauce:

Ingredients:

- 8 oz spaghetti noodles

- 1 cup raw cashews

- 1/2 cup nutritional yeast

- 1 clove garlic, minced

- 1/2 tsp salt

- 1/4 tsp black pepper

- 1/4 cup almond milk

- 1 tbsp olive oil

- Optional toppings: chopped parsley, sliced vegan bacon (such as tempeh or seitan)

Instructions:

1. Cook spaghetti noodles according to package directions. Drain and set aside.

2. In a blender, combine cashews, nutritional yeast, garlic, salt, pepper, and almond milk. Blend until smooth and creamy.

3. Heat olive oil in a large skillet over medium heat.

4. Add cooked spaghetti noodles to the skillet and pour the cashew cream sauce over the noodles.

5. Stir to coat noodles evenly and cook for another 2-3 minutes or until heated through.

6. Serve hot, topped with chopped parsley and vegan bacon if desired. Enjoy!

7. Grilled portobello mushrooms with mashed potatoes:

Ingredients:

- 4 large portobello mushroom caps
- 2 tbsp balsamic vinegar
- 2 tbsp olive oil
- Salt and pepper to taste
- 4 medium potatoes, peeled and cubed
- 1/4 cup almond milk
- 1 tbsp vegan butter
- Optional toppings: chopped fresh parsley, diced green onions

Instructions:

1. Preheat grill or a grill pan over medium-high heat.

2. In a small bowl, whisk together balsamic vinegar, olive oil, salt, and pepper.

3. Brush the mushroom caps with the balsamic mixture and grill for 6-8 minutes per side, or until tender and lightly charred.

4. Meanwhile, cook the potatoes in a pot of boiling water until tender, about 10-12 minutes.

5. Drain the potatoes and mash with almond milk and vegan butter until smooth and creamy.

6. Serve the grilled portobello mushrooms on top of the mashed potatoes and sprinkle with chopped parsley and green onions if desired. Enjoy!

8. Vegan shepherd's pie with lentils and veggies:

Ingredients:

- 4 medium potatoes, peeled and cubed
- 1/4 cup almond milk
- 1 tbsp vegan butter
- Salt and pepper to taste
- 1 tbsp olive oil
- 1 onion, diced
- 2 garlic cloves, minced
- 1 carrot, diced
- 1 celery stalk, diced

- 1 cup cooked lentils

- 1 cup vegetable broth

- 1 tsp thyme

- 1 tsp rosemary

- Optional toppings: chopped fresh parsley, sliced vegan cheese

Instructions:

1. Preheat oven to 375°F (190°C).

2. Cook the potatoes in a pot of boiling water until tender, about 10-12 minutes.

3. Drain the potatoes and mash with almond milk and vegan butter until smooth and creamy. Season with salt and pepper to taste.

4. Meanwhile, heat olive oil in a large skillet over medium heat.

5. Add onion and garlic and cook until onion is translucent.

6. Add carrot and celery and cook for another 5-7 minutes.

7. Add cooked lentils, vegetable broth, thyme, and rosemary to the skillet. Simmer for 10-15 minutes.

8. Transfer lentil mixture to a baking dish and spread mashed potatoes on top.

9. Bake for 25-30 minutes, or until the top is golden brown and crispy.

10. Serve hot, topped with chopped parsley and sliced vegan cheese if desired. Enjoy!

9. Vegan "chickn" Caesar salad with tempeh or tofu:

Ingredients:

- 1 package of tempeh or tofu

- 1/2 cup vegan Caesar dressing (or make your own with vegan mayo, lemon juice, Dijon mustard, and garlic)

- 1 head of romaine lettuce

- 1/4 cup vegan parmesan cheese, grated (or make your own with cashews and nutritional yeast)

- Croutons (optional)

Instructions:

1. Preheat oven to 375°F (190°C) and line a baking sheet with parchment paper.

2. Cut tempeh or tofu into small cubes and toss with 1/4 cup of Caesar dressing. Spread onto the baking sheet in a single layer.

3. Bake for 20-25 minutes, or until golden brown and crispy.

4. Wash and dry romaine lettuce and chop into bite-size pieces.

5. Toss lettuce with remaining 1/4 cup of Caesar dressing and top with baked tempeh/tofu, vegan parmesan cheese, and croutons if desired.

6. Serve immediately

10. Vegan Sloppy Joes with Lentils and Veggies:

Ingredients:

- 1 cup lentils, cooked
- 1 onion, diced
- 2 cloves garlic, minced
- 1 bell pepper, diced
- 1 carrot, grated
- 1 can of crushed tomatoes

- 2 tbsp tomato paste
- 1 tbsp chili powder
- 1 tsp smoked paprika
- Salt and pepper, to taste
- Hamburger buns

Instructions:

1. In a large pan, sauté onion until softened. Add in garlic, bell pepper, and grated carrot and cook for a few minutes until veggies are softened.

2. Add in cooked lentils, crushed tomatoes, tomato paste, chili powder, smoked paprika, salt, and pepper. Stir well and let simmer for 15-20 minutes.

3. Serve on hamburger buns and enjoy!

11. Vegan Sweet Potato and Black Bean Enchiladas:

Ingredients:

- 1 large, sweet potato, peeled and cubed
- 1 can black beans, drained and rinsed
- 1 onion, diced
- 2 cloves garlic, minced
- 1 red bell pepper, diced
- 1 tbsp chili powder
- 1 tsp cumin
- Salt and pepper, to taste
- 8-10 corn tortillas
- 1 can enchilada sauce
- Vegan cheese (optional)

Instructions:

1. Preheat oven to 375°F (190°C).

2. In a large pan, sauté onion until softened. Add in garlic, sweet potato, and red bell pepper and cook for a few minutes until veggies are softened.

3. Add in black beans, chili powder, cumin, salt, and pepper. Stir well to combine.

4. Warm tortillas in the microwave to make them pliable.

5. Spoon sweet potato and black bean mixture onto each tortilla and roll up tightly.

6. Place rolled tortillas into a baking dish and cover with enchilada sauce. Top with vegan cheese if desired.

7. Bake for 25-30 minutes, or until heated through and bubbly.

8. Serve hot and enjoy!

12. Vegan Eggplant Parmesan with Marinara Sauce:

Ingredients:

- 2 medium-sized eggplants, sliced into rounds
- 1 cup breadcrumbs
- 1/2 cup nutritional yeast
- 2 tsp Italian seasoning
- Salt and pepper, to taste
- 1 jar marinara sauce
- Vegan mozzarella cheese (optional)
- Fresh basil leaves

Instructions:

1. Preheat oven to 400°F (200°C) and line a baking sheet with parchment paper.

2. In a bowl, mix breadcrumbs, nutritional yeast, Italian seasoning, salt, and pepper.

3. Dip each eggplant slice into the breadcrumb mixture, making sure to coat well.

4. Place coated eggplant slices onto the prepared baking sheet and bake for 20-25 minutes, or until golden brown and crispy.

5. Pour marinara sauce into a large pan and heat over medium heat until warmed through.

6. Add baked eggplant slices to the marinara sauce and stir gently to coat.

7. Transfer eggplant slices to a baking dish and top with vegan mozzarella cheese if desired.

8. Bake for an additional 10-15 minutes, or until cheese is melted and bubbly.

9. Serve hot, topped with fresh basil leaves.

13. Vegan Mushroom Stroganoff with Tofu or Tempeh:

Ingredients:

- 1 package of tofu or tempeh
- 1 onion, diced
- 2 cloves garlic, minced
- 8 oz mushrooms, sliced
- 1 tbsp olive oil
- 1 cup vegetable broth
- 2 tbsp flour
- 1/2 cup vegan sour cream
- Salt and pepper, to taste
- Egg-free noodles

Instructions:

1. Cook noodles according to package instructions.

2. Cut tofu or tempeh into small cubes.

3. In a large pan, sauté onion until softened. Add in garlic and mushrooms and cook for a few minutes until mushrooms are cooked.

4. Remove mushroom mixture from the pan.

5. In the same pan, add olive oil and then tofu or tempeh cubes. Sauté until golden brown.

6. Sprinkle flour over the tofu or tempeh and stir for a minute.

7. Add back the mushroom mixture and pour in vegetable broth.

8. Stir until sauce thickens then add vegan sour cream.

9. Season with salt and pepper to taste.

10. Serve over egg-free noodles.

14. Vegan Creamy Tomato and Basil Soup:

Ingredients:

- 4 cups diced tomatoes
-1 onion, diced.
- 2 cloves garlic, minced
- 1 tbsp olive oil

- 2 cups vegetable broth
- 1 cup coconut milk
- 1/4 cup chopped fresh basil
- Salt and pepper, to taste

Instructions:

1. In a large pot, heat olive oil over medium heat.

2. Add diced onion and cook until softened, about 5 minutes.

3. Add minced garlic and cook for another minute.

4. Add diced tomatoes and vegetable broth to the pot.

5. Bring the mixture to a boil, then reduce heat and let simmer for 15-20 minutes.

6. Using an immersion blender or transferring to a blender in batches, blend the soup until smooth.

7. Return soup to the pot and stir in coconut milk and chopped basil.

8. Heat the soup until warmed through.

9. Season with salt and pepper to taste.

10. Serve hot with crusty bread or croutons.

15. Vegan falafel with pita bread and hummus:

Ingredients:

- 1 cup dried chickpeas
- 1 onion, chopped

- 3 cloves garlic, minced
- 1/4 cup chopped fresh parsley

- 1/4 cup chopped fresh cilantro

- 1 tsp ground cumin

- 1 tsp ground coriander

- 1/2 tsp salt

- 1/4 tsp black pepper

- 1 tbsp all-purpose flour

- Oil for frying

- Pita bread and hummus for serving

Instructions:

1. Soak the chickpeas in water overnight. Drain and rinse.

2. In a food processor, pulse the chickpeas, onion, garlic, parsley, cilantro, cumin, coriander, salt, and pepper until a coarse texture is achieved.

3. Add flour and pulse briefly until combined.

4. Form the mixture into small patties.

5. Heat oil in a large frying pan over medium heat. Fry the patties until golden brown on both sides.

6. Serve with pita bread and hummus.

16. Vegan fajitas with grilled veggies and avocado:

Ingredients:

- 1 red bell pepper, sliced

- 1 green bell pepper, sliced

- 1 yellow onion, sliced

- 1 avocado, sliced

- 2 tbsp olive oil

- 1 tsp chili powder

- 1/2 tsp ground cumin

- Salt and pepper, to taste

- 4-6 tortillas

Instructions:

1. Preheat grill or grill pan to medium-high heat.

2. In a bowl, mix olive oil, chili powder, cumin, salt, and pepper.

3. Add the sliced peppers and onions to the bowl and toss to coat evenly.

4. Grill the vegetables for 5-7 minutes, stirring occasionally,

until the vegetables are tender and slightly charred.

5. Warm tortillas on the grill or in a microwave.

6. Serve the grilled veggies on top of the warm tortillas with sliced avocado.

17. Vegan cauliflower and chickpea curry with basmati rice:

Ingredients:

- 1 head cauliflower, cut into small florets

- 1 can chickpeas, drained and rinsed

- 1 onion, diced

- 3 cloves garlic, minced

- 2 tsp ground cumin

- 2 tsp ground coriander

- 1 tsp turmeric

- 1/2 tsp cayenne pepper

- 1 can crushed tomatoes

- 1/2 cup coconut milk

- Salt and pepper, to taste

- Cooked basmati rice for serving

Instructions:

1. In a large pot, sauté onions and garlic until softened.

2. Add the cauliflower florets, chickpeas, cumin, coriander, turmeric, and cayenne pepper to the pot. Stir to coat the vegetables in the spices.

3. Add the crushed tomatoes, coconut milk and a pinch of salt. Bring to a boil, then reduce heat, cover and let simmer for 15-20 minutes or until the cauliflower is tender.

4. Season with salt and pepper to taste.

5. Serve the curry over cooked basmati rice.

18. Vegan pizza with vegan cheese, veggies, and tofu or tempeh:

Ingredients:

-Pizza dough

- Vegan shredded mozzarella cheese

- 1 red bell pepper, sliced

- 1 yellow onion, sliced

- 1 cup sliced mushrooms

- 1/2 cup crumbled tofu or tempeh

- 1/4 cup tomato sauce

- 1/2 tsp dried oregano

- 1/2 tsp dried basil

- Salt and pepper, to taste

Instructions:

1. Preheat oven to 425°F.

2. Roll out pizza dough to desired thickness.

3. Spread tomato sauce over the dough.

4. Sprinkle with vegan shredded mozzarella cheese.

5. Add sliced bell peppers, onions, mushrooms, and crumbled tofu or tempeh on top.

6. Sprinkle with dried oregano, basil, salt, and pepper.

7. Bake for 12-15 minutes, or until the crust is golden brown.

19. Vegan roasted vegetable quinoa bowl with tahini dressing:

Ingredients:

- 1 sweet potato, peeled and cubed

- 1 red bell pepper, sliced

- 1 yellow onion, sliced

- 2 cups cooked quinoa

- 1/2 cup chickpeas, drained and rinsed

- Mixed greens

- 1/4 cup tahini

- 1 tbsp honey or maple syrup

- 1 tbsp lemon juice

- 1 clove garlic, minced

- Salt and pepper, to taste

Instructions:

1. Preheat oven to 425°F

2. Spread sweet potato cubes, sliced bell pepper, and sliced onion on a baking sheet lined with parchment paper.

3. Drizzle with olive oil and sprinkle with salt and pepper.

4. Roast for 20-25 minutes, or until vegetables are tender and caramelized.

5. In a small bowl, whisk together tahini, honey or maple syrup, lemon juice, minced garlic, and a pinch of salt and pepper.

6. To assemble the bowl, divide cooked quinoa among serving bowls, top with roasted vegetables and chickpeas, and mixed greens.

7. Drizzle tahini dressing over the bowl and serve.

20. Vegan baked sweet potatoes with chickpea and spinach filling

Ingredients:

- 4 medium sweet potatoes

- 1 can chickpeas, drained and rinsed

- 2 cups fresh spinach

- 1 small onion, chopped

- 2 cloves garlic, minced

- 1 tsp ground cumin

- 1 tsp smoked paprika

- Salt and pepper, to taste

- 2 tbsp olive oil

Instructions:

1. Preheat oven to 400°F.

2. Scrub sweet potatoes and pierce with a fork several times.

3. Bake sweet potatoes for 45-60 minutes, or until tender.

4. In a skillet, heat olive oil over medium heat.

5. Add onion and garlic, sauté until softened.

6. Add chickpeas, spinach, cumin, paprika, salt, and pepper.

7. Cook until spinach is wilted, and chickpeas are heated through.

8. Cut open sweet potatoes lengthwise and spoon in chickpea and spinach filling.

9. Serve immediately.

21. Vegan lentil and vegetable shepherd's pie

Ingredients:

- 2 cups cooked green lentils
- 1 large onion, diced
- 3 cloves garlic, minced
- 2 carrots, chopped
- 2 celery stalks, chopped
- 1 cup frozen peas
- 1 tbsp tomato paste
- 1 tbsp flour
- 2 cups vegetable broth
- 2 tbsp olive oil
- Salt and pepper, to taste
- 4 large potatoes, peeled and cubed
- 1/4 cup vegan butter
- 1/4 cup unsweetened almond milk

Instructions:

1. Preheat oven to 375°F.

2. In a skillet, heat olive oil over medium heat.

3. Add onion, garlic, carrots, and celery.

4. Sauté until vegetables are softened.

5. Add tomato paste and flour, stir to combine.

6. Add vegetable broth and lentils.

7. Cook until sauce thickens.

8. Add frozen peas, salt, and pepper.

9. Simmer for a few minutes.

10. In a separate pot, boil potatoes until tender.

11. Drain and mash potatoes with vegan butter and almond milk.

12. Transfer lentil mixture to a baking dish.

13. Spread mashed potatoes on top.

14. Bake for 30-35 minutes, or until top is golden brown.

22. Vegan roasted beet and walnut salad with arugula and balsamic dressing

Ingredients:

- 4 medium beets, peeled and cubed
- 1/2 cup walnuts, chopped
- 4 cups arugula
- 1/4 cup balsamic vinegar
- 3 tbsp olive oil
- 1 tbsp Dijon mustard
- Salt and pepper, to taste

Instructions:

1. Preheat oven to 375°F.

2. Spread beets on a baking sheet lined with parchment paper.

3. Drizzle with olive oil and sprinkle with salt and pepper.

4. Roast for 25-30 minutes, or until tender.

5. In a small bowl, whisk together balsamic vinegar, olive oil, Dijon mustard, salt, and pepper.

6. In a salad bowl, mix roasted beets, chopped walnuts, and arugula.

7. Drizzle dressing over salad and toss to combine.

23. Vegan tofu and vegetable kebabs with herbed rice

Ingredients:

- 1 block extra firm tofu, drained and cubed
- 1 red bell pepper, sliced
- 1 green bell pepper, sliced
- 1 zucchini, sliced
- 1 red onion, sliced
- Salt and pepper, to taste
- 2 tbsp olive oil
- 2 cups cooked rice
- 1/4 cup chopped fresh herbs (such as parsley, thyme, and basil)

Instructions:

1. Preheat grill to medium-high heat.

2. Thread tofu, bell peppers, zucchini, and onion onto skewers.

3. Brush with olive oil and sprinkle with salt and pepper.

4. Grill kebabs for 8-10 minutes, or until tofu is lightly browned and vegetables are tender.

5. In a bowl, mix cooked rice and chopped herbs.

6. Serve kebabs over herbed rice.

24. Vegan vegetable and bean stew with crusty bread

Ingredients:

- 1 large onion, chopped
- 3 cloves garlic, minced
- 2 carrots, chopped
- 2 celery stalks, chopped
- 2 potatoes, peeled and cubed
- 1 can diced tomatoes
- 3 cups vegetable broth
- 1 can kidney beans, drained and rinsed
- 1 tsp dried thyme

Instructions:

1. In a large pot or Dutch oven, heat olive oil over medium heat.

2. Add onion and garlic and sauté for 2-3 minutes, until they begin to soften.

3. Add carrots, celery, and potatoes and cook for an additional 5-7 minutes.

4. Pour in diced tomatoes and vegetable broth and bring to a simmer.

5. Add in kidney beans and thyme, and let stew simmer

for 20-25 minutes, or until vegetables are tender.

6. Serve hot with crusty bread for dipping.

25. Vegan lentil and vegetable coconut curry

Ingredients:

- 1 onion, diced
- 3 cloves garlic, minced
- 2 carrots, chopped
- 1 bell pepper, chopped
- 1 cup diced tomatoes

- 1 can coconut milk
- 1 cup red lentils, rinsed
- 1 tbsp curry powder
- 1 tsp turmeric
- Salt and pepper to taste

Instructions:

1. In a large pot or Dutch oven, heat olive oil over medium heat.

2. Add onion and garlic and sauté for 2-3 minutes, until they begin to soften.

3. Add in the carrots and bell pepper and cook for an additional 5-7 minutes.

4. Pour in the diced tomatoes, lentils, and coconut milk, and stir well.

5. Add in the curry powder, turmeric, salt, and pepper, and let the curry simmer for 20-25 minutes, or until lentils are tender.

6. Serve hot with rice or naan bread.

26. Vegan mushroom and lentil shepherd's pie

Ingredients:

- 1 onion, diced
- 2 cloves garlic, minced
- 2 carrots, chopped
- 2 celery stalks, chopped
- 2 cups mushrooms, chopped
- 1 cup green lentils, rinsed
- 3 cups vegetable broth
- 1 tsp thyme

- Salt and pepper to taste
- 4 cups mashed potatoes

Instructions:

1. In a large pot or Dutch oven, heat olive oil over medium heat.

2. Add onion and garlic and sauté for 2-3 minutes, until they begin to soften.

3. Add in the carrots, celery, and mushrooms, and cook for an additional 7-10 minutes.

4. Pour in the lentils and vegetable broth and bring to a simmer.

5. Add in thyme, salt, and pepper, and let the mixture cook for 20-25 minutes, or until lentils are tender.

6. Preheat your oven to 375°F (190°C).

7. Transfer the lentil and vegetable mixture to a 9x13 inch baking dish.

8. Spread the mashed potatoes over the top of the mixture, and smooth out with a spatula.

9. Bake for 25-30 minutes, or until the potatoes are lightly browned and crispy on top.

10. Serve hot.

27. Vegan stuffed peppers with quinoa and veggies

Ingredients:

- 4 bell peppers, halved and seeded
- 1 cup quinoa, rinsed
- 2 cups vegetable broth
- 1 onion, diced
- 2 cloves garlic, minced
- 2 carrots, chopped
- 1 zucchini, chopped
- 1 tsp cumin
- Salt and pepper to taste
- 1 cup tomato sauce

Instructions:

1. Preheat your oven to 375°F (190°C).

2. In a large pot, bring the vegetable broth to a boil.

3. Add in the quinoa, cover, and reduce heat to low. Cook for 15-20 minutes, or until the quinoa is tender and fluffy.

4. In a separate pan, heat olive oil over medium heat.

5. Add onion and garlic and sauté for 2-3 minutes, until they begin to soften.

6. Add in the carrots and zucchini and cook for an additional 7-10 minutes.

7. Add in cumin, salt, and pepper, and stir well.

8. Mix in the cooked quinoa and tomato sauce.

9. Stuff the mixture into the halved bell peppers.

10. Place the peppers in a baking dish, and bake for 25-30 minutes, or until the peppers are tender and lightly browned on top.

11. Serve hot.

28. Vegan Thai noodle soup with veggies and tofu:

Ingredients:

- 8 oz rice noodles
- 4 cups vegetable broth
- 1 can coconut milk
- 1 medium red onion, sliced
- 2 garlic cloves, minced
- 1 thumb ginger, grated
- 2 tbsp soy sauce
- 2 tbsp red curry paste
- 1 tsp brown sugar
- 1 red bell pepper, sliced
- 1 cup broccoli florets
- 8 oz firm tofu, cubed
- 1 lime, juiced
- Fresh cilantro, chopped
- Salt and black pepper to taste

Instructions:

1. Cook the rice noodles according to the package instructions. Drain and set aside.

2. In a large pot, warm up the vegetable broth and coconut milk over medium heat.

3. Add in the red onion, garlic, and ginger. Cook until the onions are translucent.

4. Stir in the soy sauce, red curry paste, and brown sugar. Mix well.

5. Add in the red bell pepper and broccoli. Simmer for about 10 minutes or until the veggies are tender.

6. Stir in the cooked rice noodles and tofu cubes. Cook for an additional 5 minutes.

7. Remove from heat. Stir in lime juice and fresh cilantro.

8. Season with salt and black pepper to taste.

9. Serve hot.

29. Vegan sweet potato and black bean burgers with avocado mayo

Ingredients:

- 1 large, sweet potato, peeled and cubed

- 1 can black beans, drained and rinsed

- 1/2 onion, finely chopped

- 1 cup whole wheat breadcrumbs

- 1 tbsp chili powder

- 1 tsp cumin

- 1/2 tsp paprika

- Salt and pepper to taste

- 4 burger buns

- Avocado mayo (recipe below)

Instructions:

1. Preheat oven to 375°F.

2. Boil the sweet potato until soft, then mash in a large bowl.

3. Add in the black beans, onion, breadcrumbs, chili powder, cumin, paprika, salt, and pepper. Mix well.

4. Form the mixture into four patties and place on a greased baking sheet.

5. Bake for 25-30 minutes, flipping halfway through.

6. Toast the burger buns and top each patty with avocado mayo.

7. Serve and enjoy!

Avocado Mayo Ingredients:

- 1 ripe avocado

- 1/4 cup vegan mayonnaise

- Juice of 1 lime

- Salt and pepper to taste

Avocado Mayo Instructions:

1. Mash the avocado in a small bowl.

2. Add in the vegan mayonnaise, lime juice, salt, and pepper. Mix well.

3. Use as a topping for the burgers or as a dip for veggies.

30. Vegan roasted butternut squash and kale salad with maple vinaigrette

Ingredients:

- 1 medium butternut squash, peeled and cubed

- 1 bunch kale, washed and torn into pieces

- 1/2 cup sliced almonds

- 2 tbsp olive oil

- Salt and pepper to taste

- 1/4 cup maple syrup

- 3 tbsp apple cider vinegar

- 1 tbsp Dijon mustard

Instructions:

1. Preheat oven to 400°F.

2. Toss the butternut squash with 1 tbsp olive oil, salt, and pepper. Place on a greased baking sheet and bake for 20-25 minutes, stirring halfway through.

3. In a large bowl, massage the kale with 1 tbsp olive oil until it begins to soften.

4. Add in the sliced almonds and roasted butternut squash.

5. In a small bowl, whisk together the maple syrup, apple cider vinegar, Dijon mustard, and a pinch of salt and pepper.

6. Drizzle the dressing over the salad and toss well.

7. Serve and enjoy!

Condiments Recipes

1. Vegan Cilantro Lime Dressing

Ingredients:

- 1/2 cup fresh cilantro leaves
- 1/4 cup lime juice
- 1 tbsp maple syrup
- 1/4 tsp salt
- 1/4 tsp black pepper
- 1/4 cup olive oil
- 1 clove garlic, minced

Instructions:

1. Add all the ingredients to a blender or food processor.

2. Blend until smooth and creamy.

3. Taste and adjust seasoning or sweetness if needed.

4. Store in an airtight container in the fridge for up to a week.

2. Vegan Ranch Dressing

Ingredients:

- 1/2 cup vegan mayonnaise
- 1/4 cup unsweetened plain plant-based yogurt
- 1 tbsp chopped fresh dill
- 1 tbsp chopped fresh parsley
- 1 tbsp apple cider vinegar
- 1 tsp onion powder
- 1/2 tsp garlic powder
- 1/4 tsp salt
- 1/4 tsp black pepper

Instructions:

1. In a mixing bowl, whisk together all the ingredients until well combined.

2. Taste and adjust seasoning as needed.

3. Transfer to an airtight container and store in the fridge for up to a week.

3. Vegan Teriyaki Sauce

Ingredients:

- 1/4 cup soy sauce
- 2 tbsp maple syrup
- 1 tbsp rice vinegar
- 1 tsp garlic powder
- 1/2 tsp onion powder
- 1/4 tsp ground ginger
- 1 tbsp cornstarch
- 1/4 cup water

Instructions:

1. In a small saucepan, combine the soy sauce, maple syrup, rice vinegar, garlic powder, onion powder, and ginger.

2. Bring to a simmer over medium heat.

3. In a small bowl, whisk together the cornstarch and water until smooth.

4. Pour the cornstarch mixture into the saucepan and stir constantly until the sauce thickens.

5. Remove from heat and let cool slightly.

6. Transfer to an airtight container and store in the fridge for up to a week.

4. Vegan Mushroom Gravy

Ingredients:

- 1 tbsp olive oil
- 1/2 onion, chopped
- 2 cloves garlic, minced
- 8 oz mushrooms, sliced
- 1 tbsp cornstarch
- 1 cup vegetable broth
- 1 tsp soy sauce
- Salt and pepper to taste

Instructions:

1. Heat the olive oil in a skillet over medium heat.

2. Add the chopped onion and cook until softened, about 5 minutes.

3. Add the minced garlic and sliced mushrooms and cook for another 5 minutes, until the mushrooms are tender.

4. Sprinkle the cornstarch over the mushroom mixture and stir to coat.

5. Slowly pour in the vegetable broth, stirring constantly to prevent lumps.

6. Stir in the soy sauce and bring the gravy to a simmer.

7. Cook until the gravy thickens to your desired consistency, about 5-10 minutes.

8. Season with salt and pepper to taste.

9. Serve warm over mashed potatoes or your favorite vegan roast.

Mock Meats

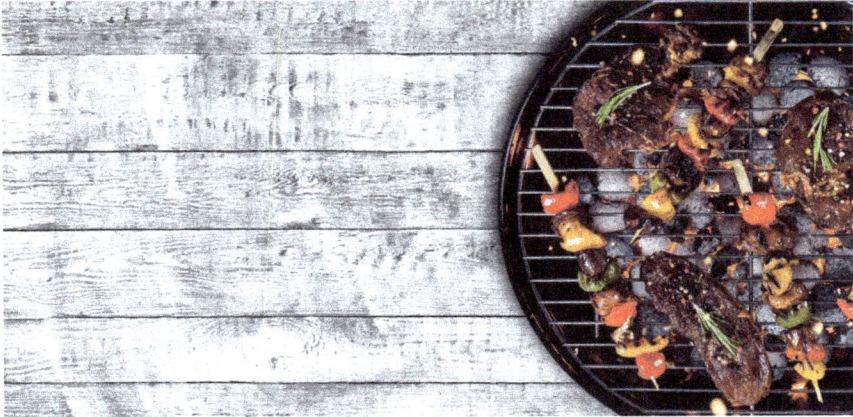

Vegan Oyster Mushroom Ribs

Ingredients:

- 2 lbs. oyster mushrooms, stemmed and sliced into "ribs."

- 1/3 cup soy sauce

- 1/4 cup maple syrup

- 2 tbsp liquid smoke

- 1 tsp smoked paprika

- 1/2 tsp garlic powder

- Salt and pepper to taste

Instructions:

1. Preheat oven to 375°F.

2. In a small bowl, whisk together soy sauce, maple syrup, liquid smoke, smoked paprika, garlic powder, salt, and pepper.

3. Place the sliced oyster mushroom "ribs" on a baking sheet lined with parchment paper.

4. Brush the marinade over the "ribs", making sure to coat them well.

5. Bake for 20-25 minutes or until the "ribs" are tender and slightly crispy.

6. Serve with your favorite BBQ sauce and enjoy!

9. Vegan Jackfruit Steak

Ingredients:

- 2 cans jackfruit, drained and rinsed
- 1 tbsp olive oil
- 1 onion, thinly sliced
- 3 garlic cloves, minced
- 1 tsp smoked paprika
- 1 tsp ground cumin
- Salt and pepper to taste

Instructions:

1. Heat olive oil in a large skillet over medium-high heat.

2. Add the sliced onion and cook until softened and lightly browned, about 5 minutes.

3. Add the minced garlic, smoked paprika, cumin, salt, and pepper. Cook for 1-2 minutes until fragrant.

4. Add the jackfruit and stir to coat it in the spices. Cook for 5-7 minutes until the jackfruit is slightly crispy.

5. Serve as a steak with your favorite sides and enjoy!

10. Vegan Seitan Sausages

Ingredients:

- 1 cup vital wheat gluten
- 1/4 cup nutritional yeast
- 1 tsp onion powder
- 1 tsp garlic powder
- 1 tsp smoked paprika
- 1/2 tsp fennel seeds

- 1/4 tsp black pepper
- 3/4 cup vegetable broth
- 2 tbsp tomato paste
- 1 tbsp soy sauce
- 1 tbsp olive oil

Instructions:

1. In a large mixing bowl, whisk together vital wheat gluten, nutritional yeast, onion powder, garlic powder, smoked paprika, fennel seeds, and black pepper.

2. In a separate bowl, mix vegetable broth, tomato paste, soy sauce, and olive oil.

3. Pour the wet ingredients over the dry ingredients and stir until a dough forms.

4. Knead the dough for a few minutes until it becomes elastic and pliable.

5. Divide the dough into sausage-sized pieces and roll each piece into a long cylinder.

6. Wrap each sausage in aluminum foil and twist the ends to secure it.

7. Steam the sausages for 30 minutes.

8. Let the sausages cool slightly before unwrapping them from the aluminum foil.

9. Heat a skillet over medium-high heat and lightly grease it with oil.

10. Cook the sausages for 2-3 minutes on each side until they are browned and crispy.

11. Serve as you would traditional sausages and enjoy!

30 Vegan Dessert Recipes

10 Vegan - 10 Sugar Free -10 Gluten Free

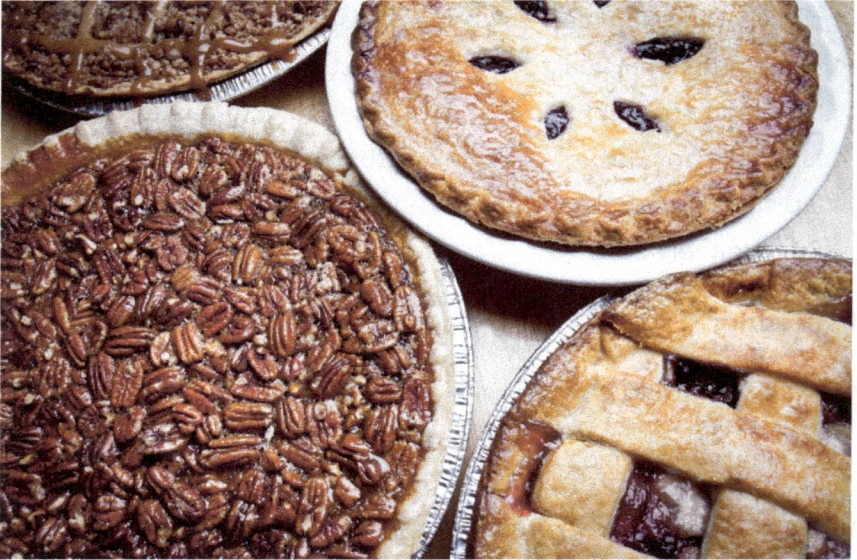

10 Vegan Dessert Recipes

1. Vegan Brownies

Ingredients:

- 1 cup flour
- 1/2 cup cocoa powder
- 3/4 cup sugar
- 1 tsp baking powder
- 1/4 tsp salt
- 1/2 cup almond milk
- 1/2 cup vegetable oil
- 1 tsp vanilla extract

Instructions:

1. Preheat oven to 350°F (175°C).

2. Combine all dry ingredients in a bowl.

3. In a separate bowl, mix almond milk, vegetable oil, and vanilla extract.

4. Add wet ingredients to dry ingredients until just combined.

5. Pour batter into greased 8x8 inch baking pan.

6. Bake for 25-30 minutes or until toothpick comes out clean.

7. Allow to cool before cutting into squares.

2. Vegan Apple Pie

Ingredients:

- 6 cups sliced apples
- 1 tsp cinnamon
- 1/4 tsp nutmeg
- 1/4 tsp allspice
- 1/4 cup flour
- 1/4 cup maple syrup
- 1 tbsp lemon juice
- pie crust (vegan)

Instructions:

1. Preheat oven to 375°F (190°C).

2. Combine sliced apples, cinnamon, nutmeg, allspice, flour, maple syrup, and lemon juice in a large bowl.

3. Roll out pie crust and place in 9-inch pie dish.

4. Pour apple mixture into pie crust.

5. Cover with another rolled-out pie crust; seal edges.

6. Cut slits in top crust for steam to escape.

7. Bake for 45-50 minutes or until filling is bubbly and crust is golden brown.

8. Let pie cool for at least 1 hour before serving.

3. Vegan Peach Cobbler

Ingredients:

- 4 cups sliced peaches
- 1/2 cup flour
- 1/2 cup sugar
- 1 tsp baking powder
- 1/4 tsp salt
- 1/2 cup almond milk
- 1/4 cup vegetable oil
- 1 tsp vanilla extract

Instructions:

1. Preheat oven to 375°F (190°C).

2. Combine sliced peaches, flour, and sugar in a baking dish.

3. In a separate bowl, mix baking powder and salt.

4. Add almond milk, vegetable oil, and vanilla extract to dry ingredients and mix until just combined.

5. Pour batter on top of peaches, spreading it evenly.

6. Bake for 40-45 minutes or until golden brown.

7. Allow to cool before serving.

4. Vegan Ice Cream Sandwiches

Ingredients:

- Vegan ice cream

- Vegan chocolate chip cookies

Instructions:

1. Scoop ice cream onto half of the cookies.

2. Cover with another cookie to make a sandwich.

3. Freeze until firm, about 1 hour.

4. Enjoy!

5. Vegan Donuts

Ingredients:

- 2 cups flour

- 1/2 cup sugar

- 1 tbsp baking powder

- 1/2 tsp salt

- 3/4 cup almond milk

- 1 flax egg (1 tbsp ground flaxseed mixed with 3 tbsp water)

- 1/4 cup vegetable oil

- 1 tsp vanilla extract

Instructions:

1. Preheat oven to 375°F (190°C).

2. In a large bowl, combine flour, sugar, baking powder, and salt.

3. In a separate bowl, mix almond milk, flax egg, vegetable oil, and vanilla extract.

4. Pour wet ingredients into dry ingredients and mix until just combined.

5. Place batter into donut pans and bake for 12-15 minutes or until golden brown.

6. Allow to cool before serving.

6. Vegan Cupcakes

Ingredients:

- 1 1/2 cups flour
- 1/2 cup sugar
- 1 tsp baking powder
- 1/4 tsp salt

- 3/4 cup almond milk
- 1/4 cup vegetable oil
- 1 tsp vanilla extract

Instructions:

1. Preheat oven to 350°F (175°C).

2. In a large bowl, combine flour, sugar, baking powder, and salt.

3. In a separate bowl, mix almond milk, vegetable oil, and vanilla extract.

4. Pour wet ingredients into dry ingredients and mix until just combined.

5. Place batter into lined muffin tins and bake for 18-20 minutes or until toothpick comes out clean.

6. Allow to cool before frosting with your favorite vegan frosting.

7. Vegan Bread Pudding

Ingredients:

- 1 loaf day-old bread (cubed)
- 4 cups almond milk
-- 1/2 cup sugar

- 1 tbsp vanilla extract
- 1 tsp ground cinnamon
- 1/4 tsp ground nutmeg

- 1/4 tsp salt
- 1/2 cup raisins

- 1/4 cup chopped nuts (optional)

Instructions:

1. Preheat oven to 350°F (175°C).

2. In a large bowl, whisk together almond milk, sugar, vanilla extract, cinnamon, nutmeg, and salt.

3. Add in cubed day-old bread, raisins, and chopped nuts (if using) and mix until bread is soaked through.

4. Pour mixture into a lightly greased baking dish.

5. Bake for 45-50 minutes or until top is golden brown and mixture is set.

6. Serve warm with your favorite vegan sauce or whipped cream. Enjoy!

8. Vegan Banana Pudding

Ingredients:

- 4 ripe bananas
- 2 cups almond milk
- 1/3 cup cornstarch
- 1/4 cup sugar

- 1 tsp vanilla extract
- A pinch of salt
- Vegan vanilla wafers

Instructions:

1. In a blender, blend 3 of the bananas until smooth.

2. In a saucepan, heat the blended banana and almond milk over medium heat.

3. In a separate bowl, whisk together cornstarch, sugar, vanilla extract, and salt.

4. Gradually add the dry mixture to the warm banana and

almond milk mixture, whisking constantly.

5. Continue whisking until the mixture has thickened, then remove from heat.

6. Layer your vegan vanilla wafers and sliced bananas in a serving dish and pour the pudding mixture on top.

7. Cover and chill in the refrigerator for at least 2 hours before serving.

9. Vegan Rice Pudding

Ingredients:

- 1 cup short-grain rice
- 4 cups almond milk
- 1/2 cup sugar
- 1 tsp vanilla extract
- 1/4 tsp ground cinnamon
- 1/4 tsp ground nutmeg
- A pinch of salt

Instructions:

1. Rinse the rice and cook according to package instructions using almond milk instead of water.

2. In a saucepan, combine sugar, vanilla extract, cinnamon, nutmeg, and salt with 1 cup of almond milk.

3. Heat over medium heat until the sugar dissolves, then pour in the remaining almond milk.

4. Stir in the cooked rice and continue cooking over low heat until the mixture has thickened.

5. Divide the pudding into bowls and let it cool.

6. Cover and chill in the refrigerator for at least an hour before serving.

10. Vegan Oatmeal Cookies

Ingredients:

- 2 cups old-fashioned rolled oats
- 1 1/2 cups all-purpose flour
- 1 cup packed brown sugar
- 1/2 cup white sugar
- 1 tsp baking powder
- 1/2 tsp baking soda
- 1/2 tsp salt
- 1/2 cup vegetable oil
- 1/2 cup almond milk

- 1 tbsp vanilla extract

- 1 flax egg (1 tbsp ground flaxseed + 3 tbsp water)

Instructions:

1. Preheat oven to 350°F (175°C).

2. In a mixing bowl, combine oats, flour, brown sugar, white sugar, baking powder, baking soda, and salt.

3. In another bowl, whisk together vegetable oil, almond milk, vanilla extract, and flax egg.

4. Pour the wet ingredients into dry ingredients and stir until well combined.

5. Scoop tablespoon-sized balls of dough onto a lined baking sheet and flatten slightly with a fork.

6. Bake for 12-15 minutes or until the edges are golden brown.

7. Allow to cool on the baking sheet for a few minutes before transferring to a wire rack. Enjoy!

10 Sugar Free Dessert Recipes

1. Chocolate Avocado Mousse

Ingredients:

- 2 ripe avocados

- 1/2 cup unsweetened cocoa powder

- 1/4 cup almond milk

- 1 tbsp maple syrup

- 1 tsp vanilla extract

Instructions:

1. Cut the avocados in half, remove the pit and scoop out the flesh.

2. Add all the ingredients into a blender and blend until smooth.

3. Chill in the fridge for at least an hour before serving.

2. Berry Chia Seed Pudding

Ingredients:

- 1/4 cup chia seeds
- 1 cup unsweetened almond milk
- 1 tbsp maple syrup
- 1/2 cup mixed berries (fresh or frozen)

Instructions:

1. Mix the chia seeds, almond milk, and maple syrup in a bowl.

2. Cover and refrigerate overnight or for at least 4 hours until the pudding has thickened.

3. Serve with the mixed berries on top.

3. No-Bake Vegan Cheesecake

Ingredients:

- 1 cup raw cashews (soaked overnight)
- 1/2 cup coconut cream
- 1/4 cup lemon juice
- 3 tbsp maple syrup
- 1 tsp vanilla extract
- 1/2 cup almond flour
- 1/4 cup melted coconut oil
- 1/4 cup chopped nuts for topping (optional)

Instructions:

1. Drain and rinse the soaked cashews.

2. Blend them in a food processor with the coconut cream, lemon juice, maple syrup, and vanilla extract until smooth.

3. Grease a springform cake tin and press the almond flour and melted coconut oil mixture onto the bottom of the tin.

4. Pour the cheesecake mixture over the base and smooth out the top.

5. Chill in the fridge for at least 4 hours before serving.

6. Top with chopped nuts before serving (optional).

4. Vegan Peanut Butter Cups

Ingredients:

- 1/2 cup natural peanut butter
- 1/4 cup coconut oil
- 1/4 cup unsweetened cocoa powder
- 2 tbsp maple syrup

Instructions:

1. Melt the peanut butter and coconut oil in a saucepan over low heat.

2. Add the cocoa powder and maple syrup and stir until smooth.

3. Pour the mixture into muffin tins lined with paper cups.

4. Chill in the fridge for at least an hour until set.

5. Chocolate Banana Ice Cream

Ingredients:

- 4 ripe bananas, frozen
- 2 tbsp unsweetened cocoa powder
- 1/4 cup almond milk

Instructions:

1. Cut the frozen bananas into chunks.

2. Blend them in a food processor with the cocoa powder and almond milk until smooth.

3. Serve immediately or freeze for later.

6. Vegan Chocolate Chip Cookies

Ingredients:

- 2 cups almond flour
- 1/4 cup coconut oil

- 1/4 cup maple syrup
- 1 tsp vanilla extract

- 1/2 tsp baking soda
- 1/2 cup vegan chocolate chips

Instructions:

1. Preheat the oven to 350°F (175°C).

2. Mix all the ingredients together in a bowl.

3. Roll the dough into small balls and place them on a baking sheet.

4. Bake for 10-12 minutes, until golden brown.

7. Strawberry Nice Cream

Ingredients:

- 4 ripe bananas, frozen
- 1 cup fresh strawberries

- 1/4 cup almond milk

Instructions:

1. Cut the frozen bananas into chunks.

2. Blend them in a food processor with the fresh

strawberries and almond milk until smooth.

3. Serve immediately or freeze for later.

8. Raw Vegan Brownies

Ingredients:

- 1 cup raw walnuts
- 1 cup pitted dates
- 1/4 cup unsweetened cocoa powder
- 1 tsp vanilla extract
- 1/4 tsp salt

Instructions:

1. Blend all the ingredients together in a food processor until smooth.

2. Line a small baking dish with parchment paper and press the mixture into it.

3. Chill in the fridge for at least an hour before slicing and serving.

9. Vegan Lemon Bars

Ingredients:

- 1 cup almond flour
- 1/4 cup coconut oil
- 1/4 cup maple syrup
- 1/4 cup lemon juice
- 1 tbsp lemon zest

Instructions:

1. Preheat the oven to 350°F (175°C).

2. Mix the almond flour, coconut oil, and maple syrup together in a bowl.

3. Press the mixture into a greased baking dish and bake for 10-12 minutes, until lightly golden.

4. Mix the lemon juice and zest together in a separate bowl.

5. Pour the lemon mixture over the baked base and bake for another 10-12 minutes.

6. Let it cool before slicing and serving. Enjoy your delicious vegan lemon bars!

10 Gluten Free Dessert Recipes

1. Chocolate Avocado Pudding

Ingredients:

- 2 ripe avocados
- 1/2 cup unsweetened cocoa powder

- 1/4 cup maple syrup

- 1/4 cup almond milk

- 1 tsp vanilla extract

Instructions:

1. Blend all the ingredients together in a food processor until smooth.

2. Serve chilled with your favorite toppings, such as fresh fruit or nuts.

2. Coconut Macaroons

Ingredients:

- 2 cups unsweetened shredded coconut

- 1/4 cup maple syrup

- 1/4 cup melted coconut oil

- 1 tsp vanilla extract

- Pinch of salt

Instructions:

1. Preheat the oven to 350°F (175°C).

2. Mix all the ingredients together in a bowl.

3. Scoop the mixture onto a lined baking sheet and bake for 12-15 minutes, until lightly golden.

4. Let the macaroons cool before serving.

3. Peanut Butter Cookies

Ingredients:

- 1 cup natural peanut butter

- 1/2 cup coconut sugar

- 1 flax egg (1 tbsp ground flaxseed + 3 tbsp water)

- 1/2 tsp baking soda

- 1/4 tsp salt

Instructions:

1. Preheat the oven to 350°F (175°C).

2. Mix all the ingredients together in a bowl.

3. Scoop the dough onto a lined baking sheet and press down with a fork to create a crisscross pattern.

4. Bake for 10-12 minutes, until lightly golden.

5. Let the cookies cool before serving.

4. Raspberry Sorbet

Ingredients:

- 4 cups frozen raspberries
- 1/2 cup maple syrup
- 1/4 cup water
- 1 tbsp lemon juice

Instructions:

1. Blend all the ingredients together in a food processor until smooth.

2. Serve immediately or freeze for later.

5. Chocolate Chip Blondies

Ingredients:

- 2 cups almond flour
- 1/4 cup coconut oil
- 1/4 cup maple syrup
- 1 flax egg (1 tbsp ground flaxseed + 3 tbsp water)
- 1 tsp vanilla extract
- Pinch of salt
- 1/2 cup vegan chocolate chips

Instructions:

1. Preheat the oven to 350°F (175°C).

2. Mix all the ingredients together in a bowl.

3. Pour the mixture into a greased baking dish and bake for 20-25 minutes, until golden brown.

4. Let the blondies cool before slicing and serving.

6. Mango Coconut Popsicles

Ingredients:

- 2 cups chopped mango
- 1 cup canned coconut milk
- 1/4 cup maple syrup
- 1 tsp vanilla extract

Instructions:

1. Blend all the ingredients together in a food processor until smooth.

2. Pour the mixture into popsicle molds and freeze for at least 4 hours.

3. Enjoy your delicious mango coconut popsicles!

7. Blueberry Crumble Bars

Ingredients:

- 1 cup rolled oats
- 1 cup almond flour
- 1/4 cup melted coconut oil
- 1/4 cup maple syrup
- 1 tsp vanilla extract
- Pinch of salt
- 1 cup fresh or frozen blueberries

Instructions:

1. Preheat the oven to 350°F (175°C).

2. Mix the oats, almond flour, coconut oil, maple syrup, vanilla extract, and salt together in a bowl.

3. Press half of the mixture into a greased baking dish.

4. Spread the blueberries on top of the mixture.

5. Sprinkle the remaining mixture on top of the blueberries.

6. Bake for 25-30 minutes, until lightly golden.

7. Let the bars cool before slicing and serving.

8. Vanilla Almond Energy Balls

Ingredients:

- 1 cup almond flour
- 1/4 cup almond butter
- 1/4 cup maple syrup
- 1 tsp vanilla extract
- Pinch of salt

Instructions:

1. Mix all the ingredients together in a bowl.

2. Roll the mixture into small balls.

3. Store the energy balls in the fridge for up to a week.

9. Chocolate Banana Ice Cream

Ingredients:

- 2 frozen bananas
- 1/4 cup unsweetened cocoa powder
- 1/4 cup almond milk

Instructions:

1. Blend all the ingredients together in a food processor until smooth.

2. Serve immediately or freeze for later.

10. Cinnamon Sugar Donut Holes

Ingredients:

- 2 cups almond flour
- 1/4 cup coconut oil

- 1/4 cup maple syrup
- 1 flax egg (1 tbsp ground flaxseed
- 3 tbsp water)
- 1 tsp baking powder

- 1/2 tsp cinnamon
- Pinch of salt
- 1/4 cup granulated sugar
- 1 tsp cinnamon

Instructions:

1. Preheat the oven to 350°F (175°C).

2. Mix the almond flour, coconut oil, maple syrup, flax egg, baking powder, cinnamon, and salt together in a bowl.

3. Roll the dough into small balls and place them on a lined baking sheet.

4. Bake for 15-18 minutes, until lightly golden.

5. Mix the granulated sugar and cinnamon together in a separate bowl.

6. Roll the warm donut holes in the cinnamon sugar mixture.

7. Serve and enjoy your tasty vegan donut holes!

CHAPTER 15:
HIDDEN ANIMAL PRODUCTS IN YOUR FAVORITE SWEET TREATS AND DRINKS

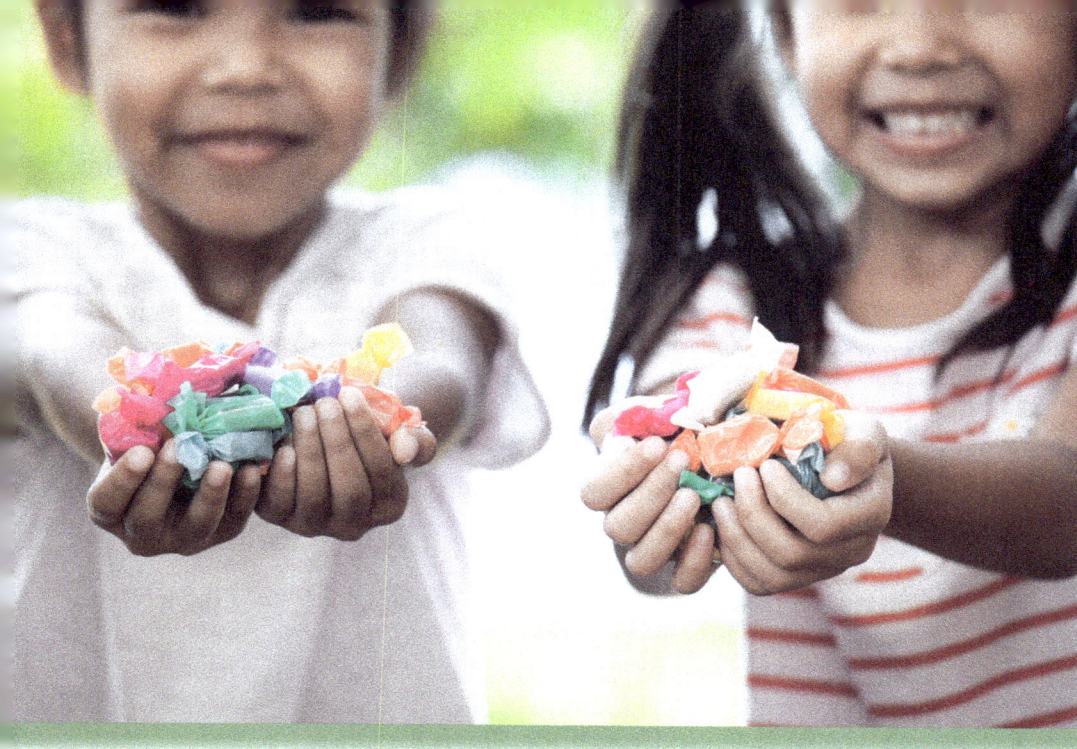

I grew up loving specific sweets. Candy in particular! My favorite was jolly ranchers and gummy bears! Sadly, as an adult/ post vegan transition I can no longer indulge. As a kid, all my friends and I would enjoy sharing the different colors since the color of the candies were associated with the flavors.

Now I simply stick to fruits! Quite boring ehhhh!

If you are like me, you're probably wondering why some candies, chips, and alcoholic beverages are not vegan-friendly?

Well, it's because many of them contain animal products that are often overlooked. These ingredients are present in many popular brands, but people remain unaware of them. In this chapter, I will shed light on the most found non-vegan ingredients and list the foods that contain them.

Beeswax: This is a natural wax produced by honeybees. Since it comes from an animal, it is not vegan.

Casein: This is a protein found in milk. Since it comes from an animal, it is not vegan.

Confectioners glaze: This is a coating used on candies and other confections. It is made from shellac, which is derived from the secretions of the lac beetle. Since it comes from an animal, it is not vegan.

Food grade wax: This can refer to various waxes used as coatings or glazes on food products. Some may be derived from animal sources (such as beeswax), making them non-vegan.

Isinglass is derived from fish bladders and is sometimes used in some wines and other alcoholic beverages to clarify them. Since it comes from an animal, it is not vegan.

Lard is a fat derived from pork. Since it comes from an animal, it is not vegan.

Vitamin D3 is typically derived from lanolin, which is found in sheep's wool. Since it comes from an animal, it is not vegan. However, some vegan alternatives for vitamin D3 are derived from lichen or mushrooms, so those would be considered vegan.

Whey is a byproduct of cheese-making, made from the liquid that remains after milk has been curdled and strained. Since it comes from an animal, it is not vegan.

L-Cysteine is an amino acid commonly used in baked goods as a dough conditioner to improve texture. However, it can be derived from both animal and plant sources. The animal-derived version is typically sourced from poultry feathers or hog hair, making it non-vegan.

Albumen, or egg white, is used as a binder and emulsifier in many candies, including marshmallows, nougats, and mints. Some chips and crackers also contain albumen. Beeswax is another surprising ingredient, which is used as a coating on candies like jellybeans and gummy bears. It is also used in lip balms and candles. Casein, a protein found in milk, is used as a flavor enhancer in some processed snacks and chips.

Cochineal extract, also known as **carmine**, is obtained by crushing female cochineal bugs and is used as a food coloring agent in many candies and drinks. Confectioners glaze, which is made from the secretions of the lac bug, is used to give a shiny finish to chocolates, candies, and gumdrops. Food grade wax, derived from insects, is used to coat fruits and vegetables, as well as certain candies and chewing gums.

Gelatin is perhaps the most well-known animal-derived ingredient in candies. It is a protein extracted from animal bones, skin, and connective tissue, used to provide texture and a gummy consistency to candies like gummy bears and fruit snacks. Isinglass, a substance obtained from fish bladders, is used to clarify alcoholic beverages like beer and wine. Lard, made from pig fat, is used in some pie crusts, baked goods, and fried snacks.

Rennet, an enzyme extracted from the stomachs of young calves, is used in cheese-making to curdle milk. Vitamin D3, which is often derived from lanolin (sheep's wool), is used as a fortifying agent in some foods and drinks. Whey, a protein found in milk, is used in some candies, chips, and protein bars to improve texture and flavor. L-Cysteine, an amino acid used to improve the texture of bread and other baked goods, is often derived from human hair or poultry feathers.

List of Non-vegan candy contains gelatin, dairy milk, or whey powder

1. Snickers
2. Kit Kat
3. Twix
4. M&M's (except for the dark chocolate variety)
5. Skittles (except for the UK and some European varieties)

6. Starburst

7. Reese's Peanut Butter Cups

8. Milk Duds

9. Butterfingers

10. Haribo gummy candies

11. Milky Way

12. Nestle Crunch

13. 3 Musketeers

14. Mars Bar

15. Hershey's Milk Chocolate Bars

16. York Peppermint Patties (contains gelatin)

17. Junior Mints (contains gelatin)

18. Tootsie Rolls (contains milk and gelatin)

19. Sour Patch Kids (contains gelatin)

20. Whoppers (contains milk)

List of Vegan-friendly candy brands and products:

1. Skittles (original variety in the US)

2. Sour Patch Kids (original variety in Canada)

3. Airheads

4. Swedish Fish

5. Twizzlers

6. Jolly Ranchers

7. Dots

8. Smarties

9. Nerds

10. Warheads

11. Vegan Rob's

12. Unreal Candy

Aside from its comparable taste there can be many health benefits to choosing vegan sweet treats. Vegan desserts tend to be lower in saturated fat and cholesterol, which can be beneficial for heart health. They may also be higher in fiber and other nutrients, like vitamins and minerals, due to the use of whole grains and plant-based ingredients. Additionally, some studies have suggested that a vegan diet can help lower the risk of certain health conditions, such as type 2 diabetes and some types of cancer. So, by choosing vegan sweet treats, you may not only be helping animals but also benefiting your own health.

When you're looking for sweet treats that are vegan-friendly, it's important to read the labels carefully.

Instead, look for sweets that are labeled as vegan or plant based. Check the ingredient list to ensure that there are no animal-derived ingredients and keep an eye out for alternatives like coconut milk or soy milk. Some vegan treats may also use natural sweeteners like maple syrup or agave nectar instead of traditional sugar. With a little bit of effort and careful label reading, you can find plenty of delicious vegan sweet treats to enjoy.

Going vegan with your sweet treats can not only benefit animals but also your health. There are some great brands out there like Enjoy Life, So Delicious, and Earth Balance that offer a range of plant-based desserts, from ice cream to cookies to cake mixes. And don't forget to check out your local health food store or vegan bakery for even more options you might find some delicious surprises!

CHAPTER 16:
VEGAN DIETS ROOTED IN CULTURAL PRACTICES

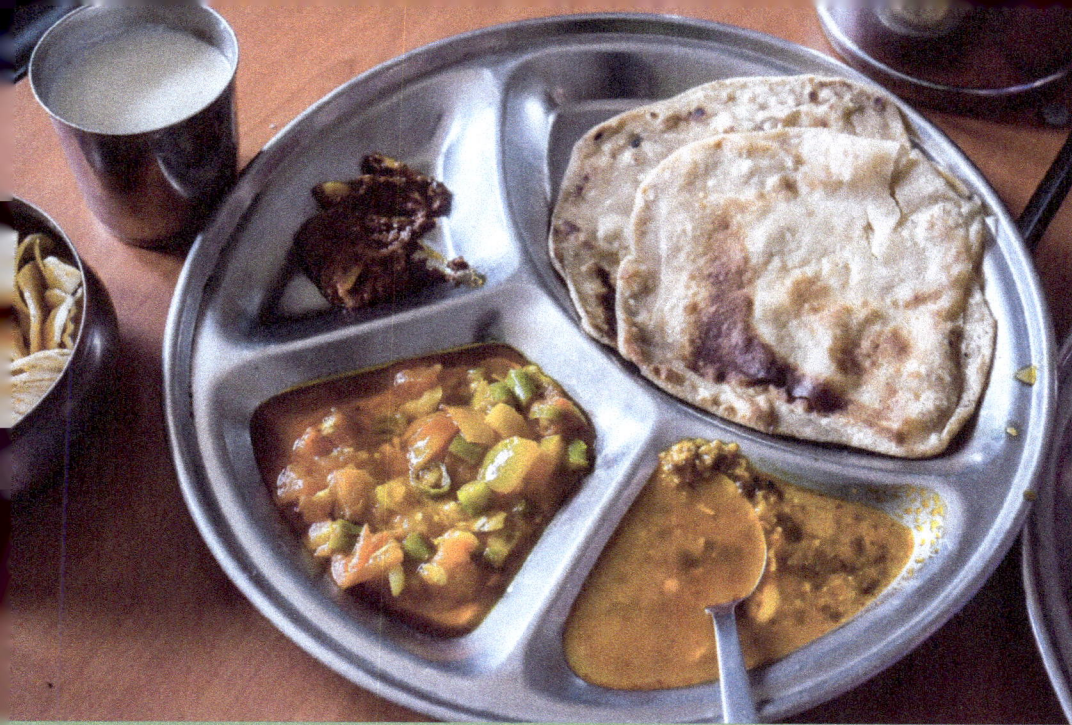

There are several vegan diets rooted in cultural practices and each culture has its own unique approach to plant-based eating, so it's a great opportunity to explore new flavors and culinary traditions. Here are some of the vegan diets I've tried over the years:

- **Indian vegan diet** - In India, there is a large population of people who follow a vegan diet due to religious and cultural beliefs. This diet includes a variety of lentils, legumes, vegetables, and grains, and is rich in spices and herbs.

- **Ethiopian vegan diet** - In Ethiopia, there is a traditional vegan diet called "fasting food" that is followed by the Ethiopian Orthodox Church. This diet includes a variety of stews and dishes made with lentils, beans, vegetables, and injera (a type of sourdough flatbread).

- **Mediterranean vegan diet -** As mentioned earlier, the Mediterranean diet can also be adapted to a vegan lifestyle by replacing animal products with plant-based alternatives.

This diet is rich in fruits, vegetables, whole grains, nuts, and olive oil.

- ■ **Buddhist vegan diet** - In many Buddhist traditions, veganism is practiced as a way of avoiding harm to animals. This diet includes a variety of plant-based foods, such as tofu, tempeh, and seitan, as well as vegetables, fruits, and grains.

- ■ **Caribbean vegan diet** - In the Caribbean, there is a variety of vegan dishes that are influenced by African, Indian, and indigenous cultures. These dishes often include staples like rice, beans, plantains, and yams, as well as a variety of flavorful spices.

The I-tal diet is a vegan diet that is rooted in Rastafarianism, a religious movement that originated in Jamaica. This diet emphasizes the consumption of natural and unprocessed foods, such as fruits, vegetables, whole grains, and nuts. It also promotes the use of herbs and spices for medicinal purposes. The I-tal diet is believed to promote physical and spiritual wellness while respecting the Earth and all living beings.

Out of the many diets I mentioned above I gravitated to the I-tal and loved it. Maybe because of my family's Caribbean roots.

Have you heard of I-tal before? Well, it's a type of plant-based diet that originated in Jamaica and is closely associated with the Rastafari movement. It was initially called "Vital" because it's "Vital for the body."

An I-tal food diet is a plant-based and natural way of eating that focuses on whole foods and excludes processed and artificial ingredients. Some of the potential health benefits of this type of diet include:

1. Improved digestion - Ital food is high in fiber, which promotes healthy digestion and can help prevent constipation.

2. Lower risk of chronic diseases - A plant-based diet has been linked to a lower risk of chronic diseases such as heart disease, diabetes, and certain types of cancer.

3. Weight management - Since Ital food is primarily made up of fruits, vegetables, and whole grains, it can aid in weight management by promoting feelings of fullness and reducing calorie intake.

4. Increased energy - The nutrients found in natural, unprocessed foods can provide sustained energy throughout the day, helping to combat fatigue and improve overall wellness.

5. Better skin health - The antioxidants and vitamins present in many fruits and vegetables can improve skin health by protecting against free radicals and promoting collagen production.

My first I-tal experience was when I decided to take a much-needed break from work and go on a vacation to Jamaica. This was my first trip to this Caribbean Island. I had always been intrigued by the country's culture, music, and of course, its cuisine. I had heard about I-tal food, which was a vegetarian diet that originated from Rastafarianism, and was curious to try it out.

On my first day in Jamaica, the resort I stayed at served various kinds of diets. Each restaurant had an I-tal menu. Each chef was thrilled to cater to my pallet and created such wonderful dishes for me. I was in heaven. As soon as I took my first bite of the first dish, I knew that this was unlike anything I had tasted before. The flavors were so fresh and authentic, and the fact that it was all grown without any artificial fertilizers or pesticides made it even more appealing to me.

Every day for the rest of my vacation, the chefs personally greeted me and created wonderful dishes. I was hooked! Each time, I was blown away by the unique flavors and freshness. It was incredible how the simplest of ingredients could be transformed into such delicious meals.

When I got back home, I couldn't stop talking about the amazing food I had eaten in Jamaica. I was so inspired by the Ital food and its health benefits that I started to incorporate its principles into my own cooking. I began sourcing local organic produce for specific ingredients and experimenting with the I-tal recipes that I had tried in Jamaica.

I was amazed at how easy it was to adopt this type of diet, and soon enough, I was sharing my experiences and recipes with friends and family. They were all impressed by the delicious meals I was making, and some even started to adopt the Ital food diet themselves.

Going on vacation to Jamaica and discovering Ital food was a life-changing experience for me. It not only opened my taste buds to new flavors, but it also inspired me to taste vegetables that I never thought I'd enjoy and incorporate them into my everyday life. Who knew that a simple vacation could have such a profound impact on my life!

So, I decided to take time and share my Ital experience with you!

There are so many cultural cuisines that incorporate plant-based ingredients in interesting and unique ways!

10 I-tal Recipes

Inspired by my trip to Jamaica.

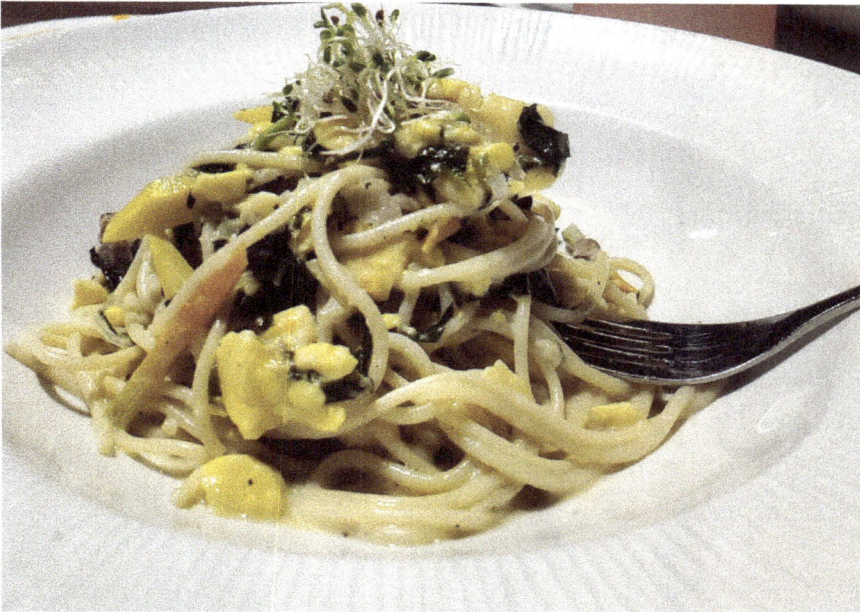

1. Ital Lentil and Vegetable Stew

Ingredients:

- 1 cup lentils, rinsed.
- 1 onion, chopped.
- 2 cloves garlic, minced.
- 1 carrot, diced.
- 1 zucchini, diced.

- 1 red pepper, diced.
- 1 can chopped tomatoes.
- 1 tsp thyme
- Salt to taste

Instructions:

1. In a large pot, sauté the onion and garlic until softened.

2. Add in the diced carrot, zucchini, and red pepper and cook for a few minutes.

3. Stir in the lentils, canned tomatoes, thyme, and salt to taste.

4. Add enough water to cover the vegetables and lentils by about 1 inch.

5. Bring to a boil, then reduce heat and let simmer for 30-40 minutes, or until the lentils are tender.

6. Adjust seasoning, if necessary, before serving.

2. Jamaican Patties

Ingredients:

- 2 cups all-purpose flour

- 1 tsp turmeric

- 1 tbsp curry powder

- 1 tsp salt

- 1/2 cup vegetable shortening

- 1/2 cup water

- 1 onion, diced.

- 2 cloves garlic, minced.

- 1 scotch bonnet pepper seeded and minced.

- 2 cups ground beef substitute (such as Beyond Meat)

Instructions:

1. Preheat oven to 375°F.

2. In a large bowl, whisk together the flour, turmeric, curry powder, and salt.

3. Cut the shortening into small pieces and use your fingers to mix into the flour mixture until crumbly.

4. Slowly add in the water, mixing with a fork until a dough forms.

5. Knead the dough on a floured surface for a few minutes, then divide into 10-12 equal pieces.

6. Roll each piece of dough into a circle about 1/4 inch thick.

7. In a separate bowl, mix the onion, garlic, scotch bonnet pepper, and ground beef substitute.

8. Spoon a little of the mixture onto one half of each circle of pastry.

9. Fold the other half of the pastry over the filling and crimp the edges with a fork.

10. Place the patties on a baking sheet lined with parchment paper.

11. Bake for 25-30 minutes until golden brown.

3. Vegan Pepper pot Soup

Ingredients:

- 2 cups diced sweet potato.
- 2 cups diced yam.
- 2 cups diced cassava.
- 2 cups okra, sliced.
- 4 cups vegetable broth
- 1 cup coconut milk
- 1 scallion, chopped.
- 1 onion, diced.
- 2 cloves garlic, minced.
- 1 tsp dried thyme
- 1 scotch bonnet pepper seeded and minced.
- Salt to taste

Instructions:

1. In a large pot, sauté the onion, garlic, scallion, and scotch bonnet pepper in a little oil until softened.

2. Add in the sweet potato, yam, cassava, okra, vegetable broth, coconut milk, thyme, and salt.

3. Bring to a boil, then reduce heat and let simmer for 30-40 minutes until the vegetables are tender.

4. Serve hot.

4. Stewed Peas and Dumplings

Ingredients:

- 2 cups cooked red kidney beans.
- 1 cup coconut milk
- 1 scallion, chopped.
- 1 onion, diced.
- 2 cloves garlic, minced.
- 1 tsp dried thyme
- Salt to taste
- 1 cup all-purpose flour
- 1 tbsp baking powder
- 1/2 tsp salt
- 1/2 cup water

Instructions:

1. In a large pot, sauté the onion, garlic, scallion, and thyme in a little oil until softened.

2. Add in the red kidney beans, coconut milk, and salt, and let simmer for 10-15 minutes.

3. In a separate bowl, mix the flour, baking powder, and salt.

4. Slowly add in the water, mixing with a fork until a dough forms.

5. Roll the dough into small balls and drop into the stew.

6. Cover the pot and let cook for 10-15 minutes until the dumplings are cooked through.

7. Serve hot.

5. Vegan Ital Spinach and Mushroom Quiche:

Ingredients:

- 2 cups sliced mushrooms.

- 2 cups spinach leaves

- 1 onion, chopped.

- 3 garlic cloves, minced.

- 1 cup coconut milk

- 3 flax eggs (mix 3 tbsp ground flaxseed with 9 tbsp water and let sit for 5 mins)

- Salt and pepper to taste

- 1 tbsp olive oil

- 1 1/2 cups whole wheat flour

- 1/2 cup vegetable shortening

Instructions:

1. Preheat your oven to 375°F (190°C).

2. In a large skillet, sauté the mushrooms, spinach, onion, and garlic until they're soft and fragrant.

3. In a large mixing bowl, combine the coconut milk, flax eggs, salt, and pepper. Mix well.

4. Add the sautéed veggies to the bowl and mix well.

5. In a separate bowl, combine the whole wheat flour and vegetable shortening. Mix until it becomes crumbly.

6. Transfer the veggie mixture to a greased quiche pan and sprinkle the crumbly flour mixture on top.

7. Bake for 30-40 minutes or until it's golden brown.

6. Vegan Jamaican Curry 'Chicken':

Ingredients:

- 1 lb. seitan, sliced.
- 1 onion, chopped.
- 2 garlic cloves, minced.
- 1 tbsp ginger, grated.
- 2 tbsp curry powder
- 1 tsp thyme
- 1/4 cup chopped scallion.
- 3 tbsp soy sauce
- 2 cups vegetable broth
- 1 cup coconut milk
- Salt and pepper to taste
- 2 tbsp vegetable oil

Instructions:

1. In a large skillet, heat the vegetable oil over medium heat.

2. Add the sliced seitan and cook until it's browned on all sides.

3. Remove the seitan from the pan and set it aside.

4. In the same pan, sauté the onion, garlic, and ginger until they're soft and fragrant.

5. Add the curry powder, thyme, scallion, soy sauce, and vegetable broth. Mix well.

6. Add the seitan back to the pan and bring everything to a boil.

7. Reduce the heat and let it simmer for 10-15 minutes.

8. Stir in the coconut milk, salt, and pepper. Let it cook for another 5-10 minutes.

7. Vegan Ital Carrot Cake:

Ingredients:

- 3 cups grated carrots.
- 1 cup raisins
- 1/2 cup chopped walnuts.
- 3 cups all-purpose flour
- 2 tsp baking powder
- 1 tsp baking soda
- 1 tsp cinnamon
- 1/2 tsp nutmeg

- 1/4 tsp cloves
- 1 tsp salt
- 1 1/2 cups sugar

- 1 cup coconut milk
- 1/2 cup coconut oil

Instructions:

1. Preheat your oven to 350°F (175°C).

2. In a large mixing bowl, combine the grated carrots, raisins, and walnuts.

3. In a separate bowl, combine the all-purpose flour, baking powder, baking soda, cinnamon, nutmeg, cloves, salt, and sugar.

4. Add the dry ingredients to the carrot mixture and mix well.

5. Add the coconut milk and coconut oil. Mix until everything is well combined.

6. Pour the batter into a greased cake pan and bake for 40-45 minutes or until a toothpick comes out clean.

8. Plantain Chips

Ingredients:

- 2 ripe plantains
- 1 tbsp olive oil

- Salt and pepper

Instructions:

Preheat oven to 400°F. Cut plantains into thin slices and toss with olive oil, salt and pepper.

Bake for about 15 minutes, flipping halfway through, until crispy.

9. Callaloo Soup

Ingredients:

- 2 cups chopped callaloo (or spinach)
- 2 cups vegetable broth
- 1 onion

- 2 garlic cloves
- 1 scallion
- 1/4 cup coconut milk

- Salt and pepper

Instructions:

In a pot, sauté onion, garlic and scallion. Add callaloo, vegetable broth, coconut milk, salt and pepper. Boil for about 20 minutes.

10. Sweet Potato and Black Bean Stew

Ingredients:

- 2 sweet potatoes
- 1 can black beans
- 1 onion
- 2 garlic cloves
- 1 scotch bonnet pepper
- 1 tbsp olive oil
- 3 cups vegetable broths
- Salt and pepper

Instructions:

In a pot, sauté onion, garlic and scotch bonnet pepper. Add sweet potatoes, black beans, vegetable broth, salt and pepper. Boil for about 20 minutes.

CHAPTER 17:
VEGANISM GROWING IN AMERICA

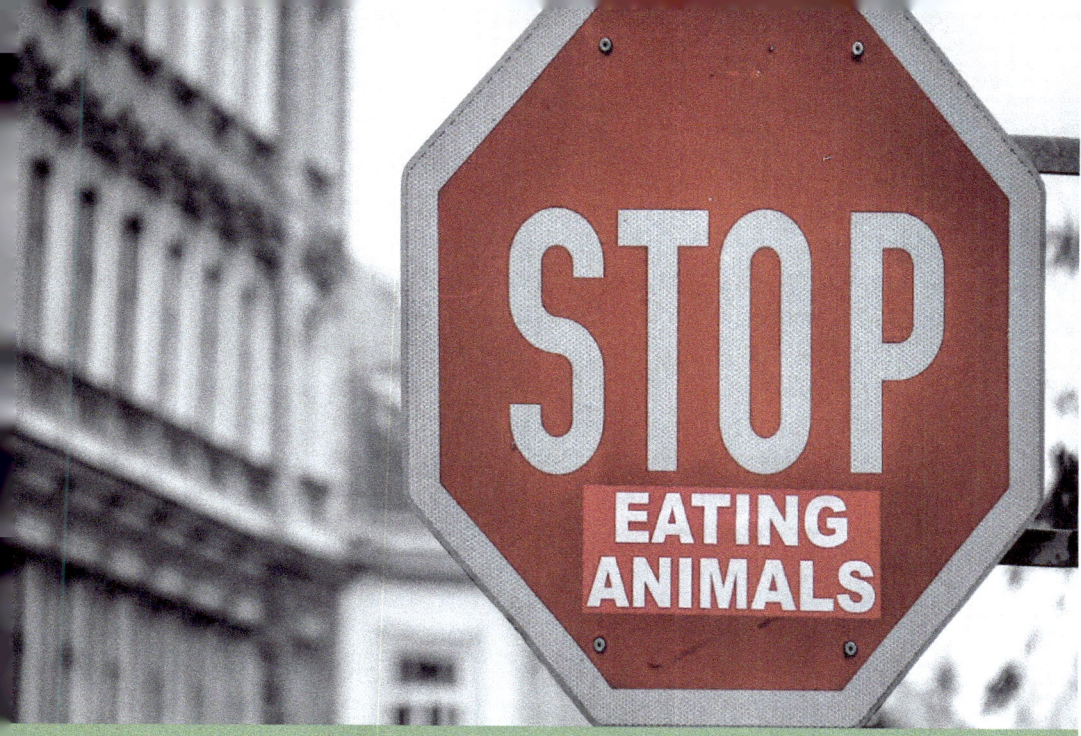

The exact number of people in the United States who follow a vegan diet is difficult to determine as there is no comprehensive data source that tracks the number of vegans in the country. What I do know is that I can start with myself and the few friends I know that are also vegan.

However, according to a 2021 report by the Plant Based Foods Association:

the sales of plant-based foods in the U.S. grew by 27% in 2020, indicating that there is a growing interest in plant-based diets. Additionally, a survey conducted by the Vegetarian Resource Group in 2020 found that 5% of U.S. adults identified as vegan, while 9% identified as vegetarian.

However, it's important to note that these numbers may not be representative of the entire population as the survey was conducted among a self-selected sample of the population.

Conducting a study on how many people in the United States are vegan would involve gathering data from various sources, such as government surveys, market research reports, and academic studies. You may also need to analyze trends and patterns in consumer behavior, as well as social and cultural factors that influence dietary choices.

One way to approach this study is to conduct a survey or questionnaire that asks respondents about their dietary habits, including whether they are vegan or follow a plant-based diet. You can administer the survey online, through social media platforms, or by mailing it to a random sample of the population.

Another approach is to analyze data from existing sources, such as the National Health and Nutrition Examination Survey (NHANES), which collects information on the health and nutritional status of the U.S. population. You can also look at market research reports that track the growth of the vegan and plant-based food industries, as well as academic studies that focus on the health and environmental benefits of plant-based diets.

The results of this study can provide valuable insights into the prevalence of veganism in the United States, as well as the factors that drive people to adopt plant-based diets. This information can be useful for businesses, policymakers, and advocacy groups who want to promote healthy and sustainable dietary choices.

CHAPTER 18:
VEGAN HUMOR: A COMPILATION OF JOKES & COMMENTS I COME ACROSS AS A VEGAN

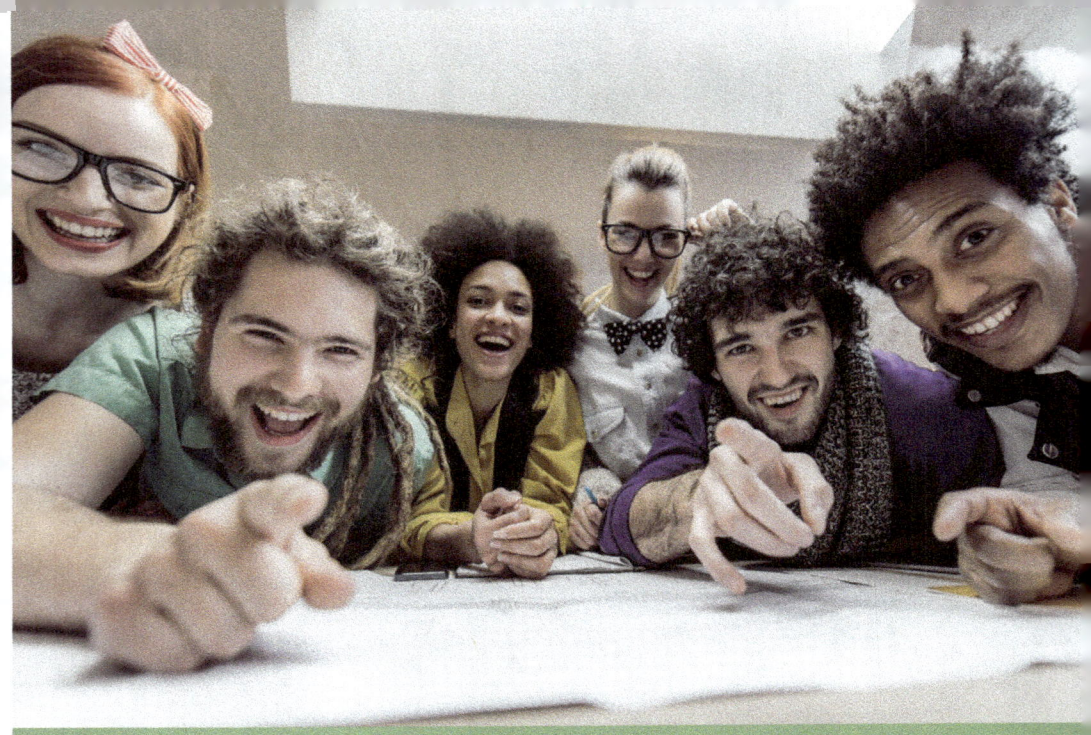

Becoming a Vegan comes with its fair share of struggles and a healthy dose of skepticism, judgements, and remarks from the world outside. To keep it light and share the funnier side of it all, I decided to compile some of the many jokes and comments I and my Vegan friends come across every now and then. Read and enjoy!

Some Comments:

- Vegans are always talking about being vegan and trying to convert others.
- Vegans are self-righteous and judgmental of non-vegans.
- Vegans only eat salads and have a boring diet.
- Vegans are weak and don't get enough protein.
- Vegans are hipsters who only care about trends and fads.

Some Jokes:

- Why did the vegan refuse to eat honey? Because it was bee-vicious!
- What do you call an alligator in a vest made of lettuce? An investigator!
- Why don't vegans eat eggs? Because they come from chickens who are always crossing the road, and nobody knows why!
- "How can you tell if someone's a vegan? Don't worry, they'll tell you, and now they'll also tell you about their WOD!"
- How do you make a vegan mani-pedi appointment? Just tofu in!
- Why did the tofu cross the road?

   To prove he wasn't chicken!

Some More:

1. What do you call a cow that's just given birth? Decaffeinated.

Explanation: Cows are often used for milk production, but in order to produce milk, they must give birth first. Decaffeinated is a play on words, as it sounds like de-calf-innated - meaning the cow is no longer producing milk.

2. Why don't vegans eat honey? Because they don't want to exploit bees.

Explanation: Veganism is not just about avoiding animal products in food, but also about respecting animal rights in general. Many vegans choose not to eat honey because they believe it exploits bees and harms their environment.

3. What's a vegan's favorite way to cook tofu? In soy-presso.

Explanation: Soy-presso is a pun on espresso, which is a type of coffee made by forcing hot water through finely ground coffee beans. Tofu is a popular plant-based protein source that can be prepared in various ways, and many vegans enjoy it in their meals.

Again, humor is very personal and what one person finds hilarious another might not find amusing at all. However, these vegan-themed jokes are a great way to poke fun at some stereotypes while also bringing a smile to someone's face.

CHAPTER 19:
TEST YOUR KNOWLEDGE

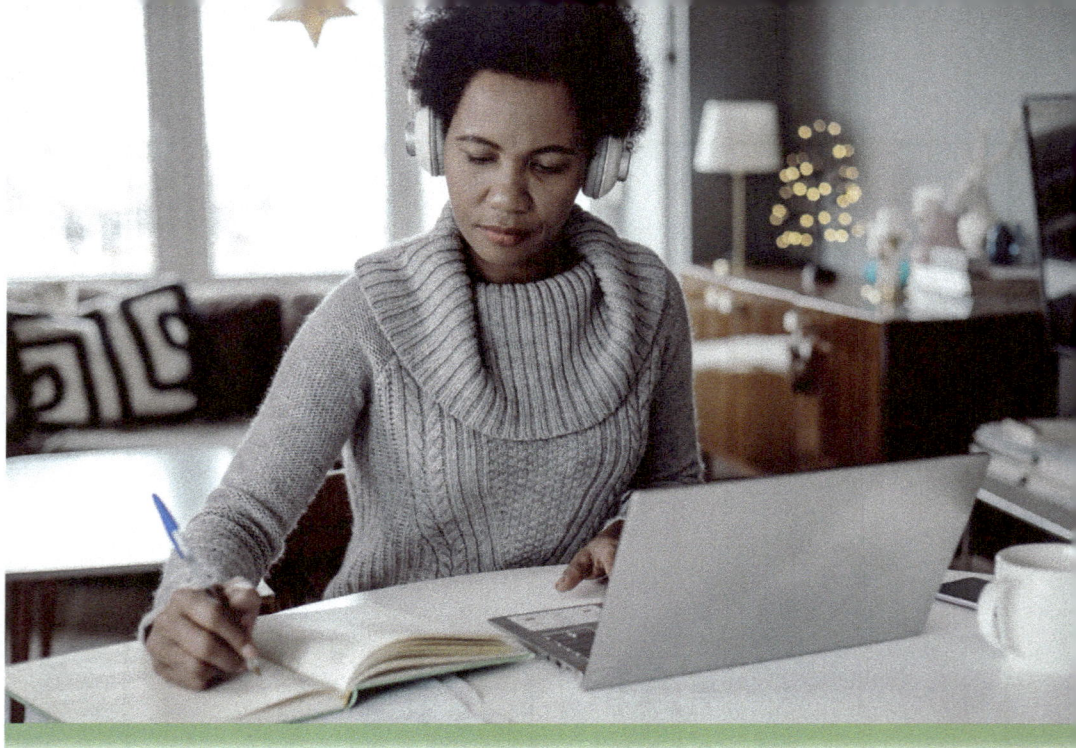

Here are 20 multiple-choice questions:

1. Which of the following is a common reason why people choose to follow a vegan diet?

a) religious beliefs

b) Ethical concerns for animal welfare

c) Health reasons

d) All of the above

2. Which of the following nutrients can be difficult to obtain on a vegan diet?

a) Protein

b) Vitamin B12

c) Iron

d) All of the above

3. Which of the following vegan-friendly foods are high in protein?

a) Lentils

b) Tofu

c) Quinoa

d) All of the above

4. Which of the following is a popular vegan substitute for cheese?

a) Cashew cheese

b) Nutritional yeast

c) Soy cheese

d) All of the above

5. Which of the following vegan-friendly foods are good sources of iron?

a) Spinach

b) Chickpeas

c) Pumpkin seeds

d) All of the above

6. Which of the following vegan-friendly foods are high in Omega-3 fatty acids?

a) Chia seeds

b) Flaxseeds

c) Hemp seeds

d) All of the above

7. Which of the following is a vegan-friendly source of calcium?

a) Almonds

b) Kale

c) Fortified plant-based milk

d) All of the above

8. Which of the following is a common ingredient in many vegan baking recipes?

a) Applesauce

b) Coconut oil

c) Aquafaba

d) All of the above

9. Which of the following is a common myth about veganism?

a) Vegans don't get enough protein

b) Vegan diets are too expensive

c) Vegan diets are low in vitamin C

d) All of the above

10. Which of the following is a vegan-friendly substitute for eggs in baking recipes?

a) Applesauce

b) Flaxseed meal

c) Banana

d) All of the above

11. Which of the following nutrients may need to be monitored on a vegan diet for optimal health?

a) Vitamin B12

b) Iron

c) Omega-3 fatty acids

d) All of the above

12. Which of the following is a popular vegan substitute for butter?

a) Coconut oil

b) Avocado

c) Nut butters

d) All of the above

13. Which of the following vegan-friendly foods are high in fiber?

a) Beans

b) Whole grains

c) Nuts and seeds

d) All of the above

14. Which of the following is a common nutrient deficiency among vegans?

a) Vitamin D

b) Calcium

c) Vitamin B12

d) All of the above

15. Which of the following vegan-friendly foods are good sources of Vitamin D?

a) Fortified plant-based milk

b) Mushrooms

c) Sunflower seeds

d) All of the above

16. Which of the following is a potential health benefit associated with a vegan diet?

a) Lower risk of chronic diseases c) Increased energy levels

b) Improved digestion   d) All of the above

17. Which of the following is a common vegan substitute for meat?

a) Tofu   c) Tempeh

b) Seitan   d) All of the above

18. Which of the following vegan-friendly foods are high in calcium?

a) Kale   c) Okra

b) Broccoli   d) All of the above

19. Which of the following nutrients should be consumed together to enhance iron absorption in the body on a vegan diet?

a) Iron and vitamin C   d) All of the concern regarding a vegan diet for pregnant above

b) Iron and vitamin D

c) Iron and vitamin E

20. Which of the following is common in a pregnant woman?

a) Inadequate protein intake   c) Lack of essential nutrients

b) Difficulty obtaining enough calories   d) All of the above

Answers to Multiple Choice Questions

1. Answer: d) All of the above
2. Answer: b) Vitamin B12
3. Answer: d) All of the above
4. Answer: d) All of the above
5. Answer: d) All of the above
6. Answer: d) All of the above
7. Answer: d) All of the above
8. Answer: d) All of the above
9. Answer: a) Vegans don't get enough protein
10. Answer: d) All of the above

11. Answer: d) All of the above
12. Answer: a) Coconut oil
13. Answer: d) All of the above
14. Answer: c) Vitamin B12
15. Answer: d) All of the above
16. Answer: d) All of the above
17. Answer: d) All of the above
18. Answer: d) All of the above
19. Answer: a) Iron and vitamin C
20. Answer: d) All of the above

Now let's see how you did!

How many did you get correct? _____

How many did you get wrong? _____

If you got less than 5 wrong great job!

CHAPTER 20:
VEGAN RESTAURANTS AROUND THE U.S

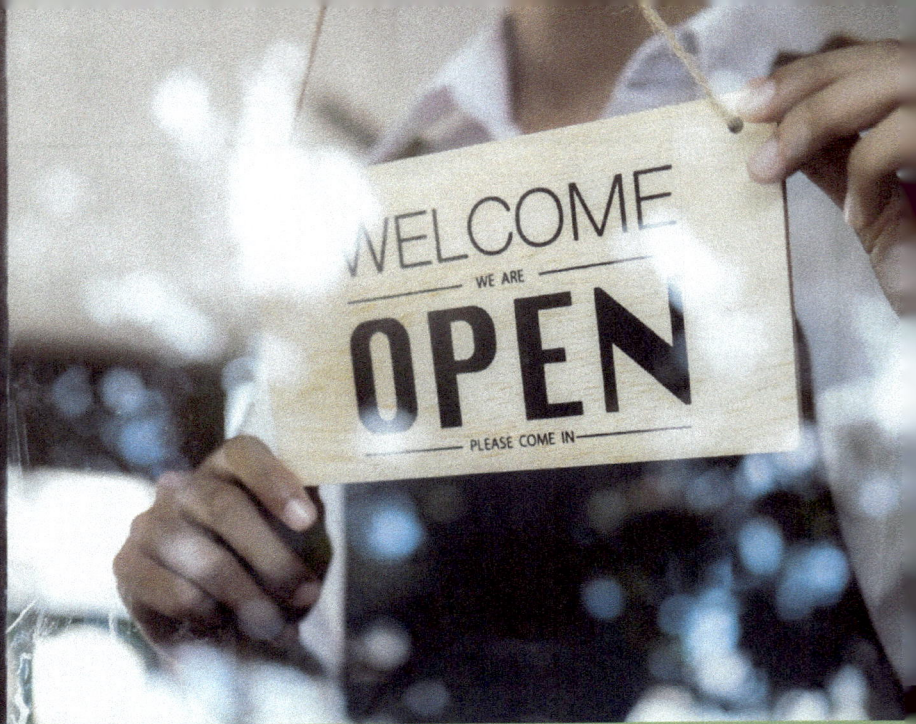

Trying vegan restaurants for the first time can be a fun and exciting experience! It allows you to explore new flavors, textures, and ingredients that you may not have tried before. You might be surprised at how delicious and satisfying plant-based meals can be.

However, it can also be a bit intimidating if you're not familiar with vegan cuisine or don't know what to order. That's why it's important to do some research beforehand and check out menus online. Some vegan restaurants even offer tasting menus or sample plates so you can try a variety of dishes in one sitting.

It's also helpful to go with an open mind and be willing to try new things! In fact, this is something that really opened a world of possibilities for me Don't be afraid to ask the server or chef for recommendations, or to make substitutions if there's something you don't like. And remember, just because its vegan doesn't mean it's automatically healthy - some vegan dishes can be high in calories, fat, or salt, so it's still important to practice moderation and balance in your diet.

Overall, trying vegan restaurants can be a great way to expand your culinary horizons and support local businesses that are committed to sustainable and ethical food practices.

Here are some of the restaurants I visited and enjoyed throughout the U.S:

New York City

1. **Candle 79** - this upscale vegan restaurant offers organic, plant-based cuisine and a wide selection of wine and cocktails. Talk about fine dining and fancy vegan food.
2. **By Chloe.** - a fast-casual vegan chain with several locations in NYC, known for their delicious burgers, sandwiches, and salads.
3. **Blossom** - a vegan restaurant with multiple locations in the city, serving up creative, gourmet dishes such as truffle mac n' cheese and seitan piccata.
4. **Avant Garden** - a small, intimate restaurant specializing in seasonal, vegetable-forward cuisine with Mediterranean influences. Very bougie.
5. **Peace food Cafe** - a casual vegan cafe with two locations in Manhattan, serving up comfort food favorites like vegan fried chicken and mac 'n cheese.
6. **Champs Diner** – Brooklyn, NY a retro-style diner serving up classic American comfort food with a vegan twist, including milkshakes, burgers, and breakfast dishes.
7. **Bunna Cafe** - an Ethiopian restaurant with a 100% vegan menu, offering a variety of flavorful stews, injera bread, and coffee. Ethnic, flavorful, and sustainable food!
8. **Modern Love Brooklyn** - a trendy vegan restaurant serving up creative, plant-based versions of comfort food favorites like mac 'n cheese, lasagna, and fried chicken.

9. **Toad Style** - a small, casual vegan spot with a changing menu of inventive dishes like buffalo cauliflower po'boys and tempeh Reubens. Inventive and quirky.

10. **Screamer's Pizzeria** - a vegan pizza joint with two locations in Brooklyn, offering delicious pies with plant-based toppings like cashew cheese and seitan sausage.

Long Island, New York

1. **3 Brothers Pizza Cafe** - This restaurant offers a wide selection of vegan pizzas.

2. **Ayhan's Shish Kebab** - Offers a variety of vegan Mediterranean dishes. All VEGAN!

3. **The Purple Elephant** - This restaurant is completely plant-based and offers a mix of cuisines including Asian and Latin. For the experimental kind.

4. **Tiger Lily Cafe** - Offers vegan options for breakfast, lunch, and dinner as well as smoothies and fresh juices.

5. **Tao's Fusion** - Offers vegetarian and vegan sushi rolls. Yes, you can be vegan and still eat sushi here!

6. **The Good Life** - This restaurant offers a variety of vegan options, including burgers, curries, and salads.

7. **Veggie Castle II** - Offers vegan Caribbean food.

8. **Phoemax** - Offers vegan pho and other Vietnamese dishes.

9. **Alem Ethiopian Village** - Offers vegan Ethiopian cuisine.

Philadelphia

1. **VEDGE** - an upscale vegan restaurant that offers inventive and flavorful dishes made with seasonal and local ingredients.

2. **Goldie** - a fast-casual restaurant in Philadelphia that specializes in falafel, hummus, and other Mediterranean-inspired dishes.

3. **HipCityVeg** - a fast-casual chain with several locations throughout Philly that specializes in vegan burgers, sandwiches, salads, and more.

4. **Bar Bombón** - a Latin-inspired vegan eatery that offers small plates, cocktails, and a brunch menu on the weekends.

5. **Charlie was a sinner** - a trendy bar and restaurant that serves up vegan small plates and cocktails in a dimly lit, intimate space.

6. **The Tasty** - a vegan diner that offers comfort-food classics like burgers, philly cheesesteaks, and breakfast dishes.

7. **Nourish Philly** – a natural healing themed, quaint, energetic, vegan comfort food that also offers vegan baked goods, sandwiches, herbs and fresh smoothies.

8. **Dottie's Donuts** - a vegan donut shop that offers a variety of unique and delicious flavors.

9. **Miss Rachel's Pantry** - a BYOB restaurant that serves up prix-fixe vegan dinners and Sunday brunches.

10. **Goldie** - a falafel-focused, fast-casual restaurant that offers a variety of toppings, sauces, and sides.

11. **Nile Café** - offers vegan plant-based soul food. We are the longest running vegan restaurant in Philadelphia.

12. **Cheezy Vegan** - 100% vegan, plant-based comfort food. Chef Reeky prides himself in using natural ingredients and local products to prepare vegan dishes in a way that vegans and non-vegans can enjoy.

13. **Uphoria Water** - Tested Alkaline water. Located in Vegan restaurants throughout Delaware and Philadelphia, PA.

New Jersey

1. **Seed Burger** - a plant-based burger joint with locations in Newark and Montclair.

2. **Veganized** - a cozy vegan cafe and bar in New Brunswick that serves up comfort food classics like mac and cheese, burgers, and pizza.

3. **Good Karma Cafe** - a vegetarian and vegan eatery in Red Bank that offers smoothies, salads, sandwiches, and more.

4. **P.S. & Co.** - an all-vegan bakery and cafe in Collingswood that specializes in gluten-free and organic options.

5. **Wildflower Earthly Vegan Fare** - a family-owned vegan restaurant in Millville that offers a variety of global cuisine, including Jamaican, Mexican, and Italian-inspired dishes.

6. **Soulful Sparrow** - a vegan cafe and juice bar in Asbury Park that offers smoothies, salads, and sandwiches.

7. **The Cinnamon Snail** - a popular vegan food truck that offers creative sandwiches, burgers, and pastries at various locations throughout the state.

8. **Animo Juice** - a healthy quick-service restaurant in Cape May that offers quinoa bowls, salads, and smoothies.

9. **Veggie Heaven** - a vegetarian and vegan Asian restaurant with several locations throughout the state, including Denville and Montclair.

10. **Grateful Plate** - a vegan meal delivery service based in Haddon Township that offers weekly meal plans and catering services.

Delaware

1. **Drop Squad Kitchen** - a vegan soul food restaurant in Wilmington that offers dishes like mac and cheese, BBQ ribs, and collard greens.

2. **Daily Veg** - is a fast casual 100% Plant Based Vegan Restaurant that offers Burger, Sandwiches, Milkshakes, Acai bowls, Smoothies and other vegan items.

3. **Ulysses American Gastropub** - a pub in Wilmington that has many vegan options, such as peanut butter and jelly wings and cauliflower steak.

4. **Juice Joint Cafe** - a juice bar and cafe in Wilmington that offers smoothies, salads, and wraps.

5. **Green Box Kitchen** - a vegan restaurant in Wilmington that offers plant-based burgers, sandwiches, and tacos.

6. **Drip café** - a Cafe in Hockessin that has vegan options, such as avocado toast and veggie burgers.

7. **Cosmic Cafe** - a vegetarian restaurant in Rehoboth Beach that has many vegan options, such as tempeh Reubens and black bean burgers.

8. **Go Vegan Philly**- a Soul food style vegan restaurant in Wilmington that offers dishes fried cauliflower, mac n cheez, cornbread and collard greens.

Georgia

1. **Cafe Sunflower** - This restaurant offers an extensive menu of vegan and vegetarian options, including salads, sandwiches, and entrees.

2. **Herban Fix** - Offers vegan dishes with Asian and American influences.

3. **Viva La Vegan** - Offers vegan comfort food such as burgers and mac and cheese.

4. **Dulce Vegan Bakery & Cafe** - Offers vegan baked goods and coffee.

5. **Tassili's Raw Reality** - Offers raw vegan dishes like wraps and bowls.

6. **Loving Hut** - A global chain of vegan restaurants offering a variety of cuisines such as Asian and American.

7. **Slutty Vegan** - offers a variety of plant-based burgers, sandwiches, and unique side dishes like vegan lobster mac and cheese and sweet potato fries.

8. **The Southern V** - Offers vegan soul food dishes such as fried "chicken" sandwiches and collard greens.

9. **R. Thomas Deluxe Grill** - Offers a wide selection of vegan and vegetarian options, including smoothies and juices.

10. **Go Vegetarian** - Offers vegan soul food dishes like BBQ ribs and mac and cheese.

Maryland

1. **Great Sage** - Located in Clarksville, this restaurant serves organic, locally sourced vegan cuisine with a variety of options for brunch, lunch, and dinner.

2. **Grind House Juice Bar** - This Baltimore-based juice bar offers fresh cold-pressed juices, smoothies, acai bowls, salads, and wraps.

3. **Pure Wine Cafe** - Located in Ellicott City, this cafe serves vegan and vegetarian dishes along with a vast selection of organic wines.

4. **The Land of Kush** - A popular vegan spot in Baltimore that offers a range of soul food-inspired dishes like vegan crab cakes, mac and cheese, and collard greens.

5. **NuVegan Cafe** - With locations in Silver Spring and College Park, NuVegan Cafe serves 100% vegan comfort foods like burgers, sandwiches, wings, and milkshakes.

6. **Roots Market Cafe** - Located in Olney, this cafe serves vegan and vegetarian dishes made from locally sourced, organic ingredients.

7. **Sticky Rice** - This Baltimore-based sushi restaurant has a vegan menu section with creative rolls like the Vegan Dragon Roll and Spicy Vegan Spider Roll.

8. **The Greenhouse Cafe** - Located in Columbia, this cafe serves vegan and gluten-free breakfast sandwiches, wraps, salads, and smoothies.

9. **Busboys and Poets** - With locations in Hyattsville and Takoma Park, this cafe/restaurant hosts open mic nights, book talks, and art shows while serving a range of vegan and vegetarian options like tofu scramble and lentil soup.

10. **Smokehouse Live** - Located in Leesburg, Virginia, this BBQ joint has a separate vegan menu section with smoked jackfruit, vegan sausages, and tempeh ribs.

Virginia

1. **Loving Hut** - With locations in Falls Church, Fairfax, and Richmond, Loving Hut serves vegan Asian-inspired dishes like noodle soups, stir-fries, and vegan sushi.

2. **Sticks Kebob Shop** - This Charlottesville-based restaurant offers a vegan kebab plate with marinated tofu, grilled veggies, and rice pilaf.

3. **The Greenhouse Kitchen** - Located in Norfolk, this cafe serves vegan and gluten-free options like smoothie bowls, avocado toast, and veggie wraps.

4. **Saadia's Juicebox & Yoga Bar** - Located in Richmond, Saadia's is a juice bar and yoga studio that also offers vegan salads, quinoa bowls, and raw desserts.

5. **Plant No. 1** - This Richmond-based restaurant serves vegan comfort food like mac and cheese, BBQ jackfruit, and fried "chicken" sandwiches.

6. **The Simple Greek** - With locations in Chesapeake and Virginia Beach, The Simple Greek offers a vegan falafel wrap with hummus, veggies, and tzatziki sauce.

7. **Peking Gourmet Inn** - This Falls Church-based Chinese restaurant has a vegan menu section with dishes like sesame tofu and sautéed mixed vegetables.

8. **Bangkok Garden** - Located in Alexandria, Bangkok Garden serves vegan Thai curries, noodle dishes, and stir-fries.

9. **Bocata Latin Grill** - With locations in Blacksburg and Roanoke, Bocata offers a vegan sandwich with marinated tofu, avocado, and plantains.

10. **Barley Mac** - This Arlington-based restaurant has a separate vegan menu section with dishes like roasted mushroom risotto and spicy lentil soup.

Washington D.C

1. **Shouk** - Located in both DC and Arlington, this restaurant specializes in plant-based Middle Eastern Street food.

2. **HipCityVeg** - With locations in Dupont Circle and Chinatown, HipCityVeg serves vegan burgers, sandwiches, and salads.

3. **Fare Well** - This DC restaurant offers vegan comfort food like mac and cheese, burgers, and brunch items.

4. **The Fancy Radish** - A vegetable-focused restaurant in DC, The Fancy Radish offers dishes like carrot sliders and smoked rutabaga "pastrami."

5. **Pow Pow** - With locations in both DC and Arlington, this restaurant serves vegan takes on Chinese and Korean street food.

6. **Equinox** - This upscale DC restaurant offers a vegan tasting menu that changes seasonally.

7. **Busboys and Poets** - With several locations in the DC area, Busboys and Poets offers a variety of vegan options including Jamaican jerk tofu and black bean chili.

8. **Evolve Vegan Restaurant** - Located in Takoma Park, Maryland (just outside of DC), Evolve serves vegan dishes like seitan piccata and stuffed peppers.

9. **Sticky Fingers Sweets & Eats** - This popular DC bakery offers vegan pastries, cakes, and sandwiches.

10. **NuVegan Café** - With locations in DC and Maryland, Nu-Vegan offers vegan soul food like fried "chicken" and BBQ ribs.

11. **Planta** – Bethesda MD, Asian-influenced. serving a menu of hits like vegan sushi, fresh juice cocktails, pasta blan-keted with a rich and spicy rosé vodka sauce, plus a veg-an version of Maryland's iconic crab dip made with fresh hearts of palm.

Charlotte, NC

1. **Bean Vegan Cuisine** - This restaurant in the Plaza Mid-wood neighborhood offers a menu of vegan comfort food like burgers, mac & cheese, and BBQ pulled pork.

2. **Living Kitchen** - This vegan and raw food restaurant has two locations in Charlotte and offers a menu of fresh and healthy dishes like wraps, salads, and smoothies.

3. **Fern, Flavors from the Garden** - This upscale vegetarian restaurant in the Dilworth neighborhood offers a menu that is mostly vegan-friendly, with dishes like mushroom risotto, seitan schnitzel, and carrot cake.

4. **Veltree** - This vegan soul food restaurant in the University City neighborhood offers a menu of southern staples like collard greens, black-eyed peas, and sweet potato pie.

5. **Luna's Living Kitchen** - This cafe in South End offers a menu of plant-based dishes that are mostly raw and organ-ic, including soups, salads, and wraps.

6. **B Good** - This chain has one location in Charlotte and offers customizable bowls and salads with several vegan options.

7. **Zizi's Vegan Takeout** - This takeout-only spot in the Plaza Midwood neighborhood offers a menu of vegan comfort food like mac & cheese, burgers, and fried chicken.

8. **NuVegan Cafe** - This chain has one location in Charlotte and offers a menu of vegan soul food like BBQ ribs, mac & cheese, and collard greens.

9. **The Greener Apple** - This vegan cafe in the Ballantyne area offers a menu of sandwiches, wraps, salads, and smoothies.

10. **Empower Raw Cafe** - This raw food cafe in the Plaza Midwood neighborhood offers a menu of juices, smoothies, and light bites like avocado toast and raw sushi rolls.

Florida

1. **Plant Miami** - This upscale vegan restaurant in the Wynwood neighborhood serves organic, plant-based cuisine with global influences.

2. **Love Life Cafe** - This vegan cafe in the Design District offers a menu of smoothies, bowls, sandwiches, and more.

3. **Bunnie Cakes** - This bakery in Wynwood specializes in vegan and gluten-free desserts, including cupcakes, cakes, and donuts.

4. **Full Bloom** - This vegan fine dining restaurant in Miami Beach offers a seasonal menu of farm-to-table dishes.

5. **Choices Cafe** - This local chain has several locations throughout Miami and offers a menu of vegan burgers, wraps, bowls, and more.

6. **Manna Life Food** - This vegan and organic cafe in Downtown Miami offers raw and cooked dishes, plus smoothies and juices.

7. **Della Bowls** - This casual eatery in the Upper East Side offers vegan and vegetarian bowls made with locally sourced ingredients.

8. **The Last Carrot** - This vegetarian and vegan cafe in Coconut Grove has been a Miami staple for over 40 years, serving up healthy eats and juices.

9. **Holi Vegan Kitchen** - This vegan restaurant in North Miami Beach specializes in plant-based versions of Indian dishes.

10. **Veganaroma** - This vegan Italian restaurant in South Beach offers pizza, pasta, and more.

California

1. **Hart House** - serves a variety of plant-based dishes, including salads, sandwiches, soups, and entrees. Some popular menu items include their vegan burger with sweet potato fries, quinoa and vegetable stir-fry, and lentil soup. They also offer vegan desserts such as chocolate cake and coconut milk ice cream. Several Locations; Westchester, Monravia, Los Angeles

2. **Gracias Madre** - This vegan Mexican restaurant in the Mission District offers dishes like plantain empanadas and mushroom tamales.

3. **Shizen Vegan Sushi Bar & Izakaya** - Located in the Mission District, this innovative sushi spot features creative vegan rolls and hot dishes.

4. **The Butcher's Son** - This vegan deli in Berkeley (just across the Bay from San Francisco) serves up sandwiches, burgers, and vegan charcuterie.

5. **Ananda Fuara** - This vegetarian restaurant in Civic Center offers a wide variety of vegan options, including lentil shepherd's pie and vegan lasagna.

6. **Seed + Salt** - This Marina District spot specializes in clean, healthy food like bowls, salads, and sandwiches.

7. **Udupi Palace** - This South Indian restaurant in the Mission District has a huge selection of vegetarian and vegan dishes, like dosas and curries.

8. **Nourish Cafe** - With locations in the Inner Richmond and Nob Hill neighborhoods, nourish offers vegan breakfast items, bowls, and salads.

9. **Loving Hut** - This chain of vegan restaurants has a location in the Sunset District, serving up Asian-inspired dishes like pad thai and curry.

10. **Citizen Fox** - This bar/restaurant in the Mission District offers vegan comfort food like mac and cheese and buffalo cauliflower wings.

11. **Wildseed** - This vegan cafe in Cow Hollow serves brunch items, bowls, and seasonal dishes.

Washington

1. **Plum Bistro -** This restaurant in Capitol Hill offers a menu of vegan comfort food like mac & cheese and BBQ tofu, as well as creative plant-based dishes.

2. **No Bones Beach Club** - This vegan tiki bar in Ballard offers a menu of tropical-inspired dishes like jerk jackfruit tacos and coconut ceviche.

3. **Cafe Flora** - This vegetarian restaurant in Madison Valley offers a menu of creative plant-based dishes that showcase local and seasonal ingredients.

4. **Frankie & Jo's** - This ice cream shop in Capitol Hill offers a menu of vegan ice cream flavors made with cashew milk and coconut milk.

5. **Wayward Vegan Cafe** - This diner-style restaurant in the University District offers a menu of hearty vegan breakfast options and classic American fare.

6. **Harvest Beat** - This fine dining restaurant in Wallingford offers a multi-course vegan tasting menu that highlights local and organic ingredients.

7. **Araya's Place** - This Thai restaurant has multiple locations in Seattle and offers a menu of vegan versions of traditional dishes like pad thai and green curry.

8. **Pizza Pi Vegan Pizzeria** - This pizzeria in the University District offers a menu of vegan pizzas made with cashew cheese and creative toppings.

9. **Cycle Dogs** - This food truck offers vegan hot dogs made with soy and tempeh, as well as vegan poutine and loaded fries.

10. **Fictitious Vegan Eats** - This food truck offers a menu of vegan versions of classic American comfort food like Philly cheesesteaks and Reuben sandwiches.

Chicago

1. **The Chicago Diner -** This classic vegetarian spot has been serving vegan comfort food for over 30 years.

2. **Native Foods Cafe** - With multiple locations in the city, this fast-casual chain offers fresh and flavorful vegan fare.

3. **Karyn's Cooked** - This cozy restaurant in Lincoln Park has an extensive menu of plant-based dishes, including plenty of gluten-free options.

4. **Upton's Breakroom** - Located in West Town, this casual eatery features a range of vegan sandwiches, salads, and sides.

5. **Kal'ish** - This counter-service spot in Uptown serves vegan breakfast items, burgers, and more.

6. **Ground Control** - This Lakeview bar and restaurant offers vegan takes on classic pub fare, as well as an impressive beer selection.

7. **Amitabul -** This Korean restaurant in Rogers Park specializes in vegan versions of traditional dishes like bibimbap and spicy tofu soup.

8. **Veggie Grill** - Another California-based chain with locations in Chicago, Veggie Grill offers a wide variety of vegan comfort food favorites.

9. **Kitchen 17** - This all-vegan pizzeria in Lakeview serves up creative pies and offers vegan versions of classic Italian dishes.

10. **Handlebar** - This Wicker Park staple serves vegetarian and vegan pub food, including a great brunch menu on weekends.

California

1. **Crossroads Kitchen** - This upscale restaurant in West Hollywood serves creative vegan dishes in a chic atmosphere.
2. **Sage Vegan Bistro** - With locations in Culver City, Echo Park, and Pasadena, Sage offers an extensive menu of vegan comfort food favorites.
3. **Shojin** - Located in Little Tokyo, Shojin specializes in vegan sushi and other Japanese dishes.
4. **Gracias Madre** - This trendy West Hollywood spot serves up Mexican-inspired vegan fare, including delicious boozy cocktails.
5. **Cafe Gratitude** - With locations in Larchmont, Venice, and Arts District, this popular vegan chain serves up fresh, locally sourced ingredients in a positive environment.
6. **Real Food Daily** - With two locations in West Hollywood and Pasadena, Real Food Daily is a longtime vegan staple in the LA dining scene.
7. **Eat Drink Vegan** - This annual festival brings together dozens of vegan food vendors from around the LA area for a day of feasting and fun.
8. **Mohawk Bend** - This Echo Park beer bar features an extensive menu of vegan pub fare, including pizzas, burgers, and more.
9. **Little Pine** - This stylish silver Lake restaurant is owned by musician Moby and features a menu of vegan dishes with Mediterranean and American influences.
10. **Pura Vita** - This West Hollywood eatery serves up inventive Italian-inspired vegan dishes, including house-made pastas.

11. **SunCafe Organic** - Located in Studio City, SunCafe serves organic, plant-based dishes with an emphasis on health and wellness.

12. **Vinh Loi Tofu** - This vegan Vietnamese restaurant has locations in Reseda and Sherman Oaks and serves up flavorful tofu dishes.

13. **The Butcher's Daughter** - This Venice restaurant features an all-vegan menu of colorful dishes made with locally sourced ingredients.

14. **Plant Food + Wine** - This Venice restaurant from chef Matthew Kenney serves up elegant, plant-based dishes in a beautiful outdoor setting.

15. **M Cafe** - With locations in Beverly Hills, Hollywood, and Brentwood, M Cafe offers a range of vegan dishes with Japanese and macrobiotic influences.

CHAPTER 21:
BE PROUD OF YOURSELF

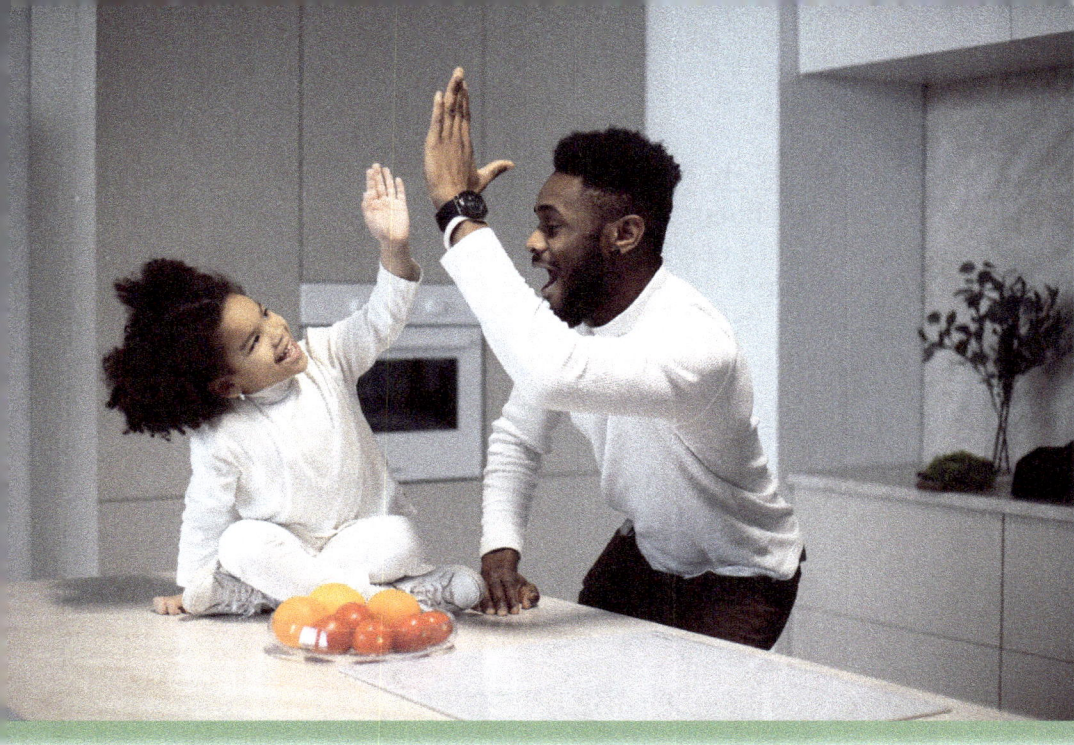

As someone who adopted and fully transitioned into a vegan lifestyle and has been actively advocating for the same – one of the most important reminders and advice I can give you is to be proud of yourself.

This shift has its psychological implications as well and people who tend to keep themselves motivated, constantly encourage themselves, and celebrate small milestones are the ones who end up staying steadfast and consistent with this too. Following are some practices to repeat:

1. **Celebrate your accomplishments:**

    It's important to recognize and celebrate all the positive changes you've made throughout your vegan journey. Take a moment to reflect on how far you've come and pat yourself on the back for making the commitment to live a healthier and more ethical lifestyle.

2. **Focus on the benefits:**

   Remind yourself of all the benefits of being vegan, such as improved health, reduced environmental impact, and animal welfare. By focusing on these positive aspects, you'll be more motivated to stick with your new lifestyle in the long run.

3. **Plan for success:**

   As you transition to a vegan lifestyle, it's important to plan for success. This may involve learning new recipes, finding new restaurants to try, or joining a community of like-minded individuals. By planning, you'll be more likely to stay on track and achieve your goals.

4. **Be patient and kind to yourself:**

   Transitioning to a vegan lifestyle can be challenging, and it's important to be patient and kind to yourself throughout the process. Remember that it's okay to make mistakes or slip up occasionally – what's important is that you keep moving forward towards your goal.

5. **Keep learning and growing:**

   Being vegan is a journey, not a destination. There is always more to learn and discover, so don't be afraid to continue exploring new foods, recipes, and ways of living. By staying open-minded and curious, you'll continue to grow and evolve as a vegan.

CHAPTER 22:
VEGAN TERMINOLOGY

1. **Vegan** - a person who does not consume or use any animal products.

2. **Plant-based** - a diet that is centered on whole, unprocessed plant foods.

3. **Cruelty-free** - products that have not been tested on animals.

4. **Ethical** - a way of living that prioritizes respect and compassion for all living beings.

5. **Meat substitute** - a food product designed to imitate meat in taste, texture, and appearance.

6. **Dairy-free** - products that do not contain dairy or lactose.

7. **Veganism** - the practice of living a lifestyle that avoids the use of animal products in all aspects, including food, clothing, and personal care items.

8. **Plant-based protein** - sources of protein that come from plant foods, such as beans, nuts, and seeds.

9. **Non-dairy milk** - plant-based alternatives to milk, such as soy milk or almond milk.

10. **Tofu** - a plant-based protein source made from soybeans that can be used in a variety of dishes.

11. **Seitan** - a meat substitute made from wheat gluten that is often used to create meat-like textures in vegan dishes.

12. **Vegan-friendly** - products or services that do not contain animal products or support animal exploitation.

13. **Nutritional yeast** - a yeast-based product that provides a cheesy flavor and is often used as a plant-based alternative to cheese.

14. **Tempeh** - a plant-based protein source made from fermented soybeans that can be used in a variety of dishes.

15. **Jackfruit** - a fruit that has a meat-like texture and is often used as a meat substitute.

16**. Aquafaba** - the liquid from a can of chickpeas that can be used as an egg substitute in recipes.

17. **Vegan leather** - a synthetic material that is used as an alternative to animal leather in clothing and accessories.

18. **Veganic farming** - a method of farming that avoids the use of animal products, such as manure or bone meal, and relies on plant-based fertilizers instead.

19. **Flax Egg:** a vegan substitute for eggs in baking recipes. It is made by mixing 1 tablespoon of ground flaxseed with 3 tablespoons of water and allowing it to sit for a few minutes until it becomes gel-like in texture. This mixture can then be used in place of one egg in a recipe.

20. **Vegan substitutes** There are several vegan substitutes for eggs in baking recipes. Some common options include applesauce, mashed bananas, silken tofu, yogurt, and vinegar mixed with baking powder. Each substitute may work differently based on the recipe and desired outcome, so it's important to experiment and find the best option for each situation.

CHAPTER 23:
HELPFUL RESOURCES

Vegan Websites

There are many great websites for vegan information, depending on what you're looking for. Here are some that helped me the most:

- **The Vegan Society:** This website offers a wealth of information on veganism, including recipes, nutrition advice, and resources for transitioning to a plant-based lifestyle.

- **PETA:** People for the Ethical Treatment of Animals (PETA) is a well-known animal advocacy group that promotes veganism as the best way to protect animals from harm. Their website offers a variety of resources on vegan living, including recipes, shopping guides, and educational materials.

- **Vegan Outreach:** This organization works to promote veganism through grassroots outreach and education. Their website offers a variety of resources for those interested in learning more about veganism, including a free starter guide and tips for eating vegan on a budget.

- **HappyCow:** This website is a great resource for finding vegan-friendly restaurants and stores in your area, no matter where you are in the world. They also offer reviews and ratings from other users, making it easier to find the best options.

- **One Green Planet:** This website is dedicated to promoting sustainable living, including veganism. They offer a variety of resources on plant-based living, including recipes, product reviews, and environmental news.

www.Eatingourfuture.com

www.summerveg.com

www.mercyforanimals.org

There are many excellent resources available online for anyone interested in learning more about veganism or adopting a plant-based lifestyle. Whether you're looking for recipes, nutrition advice, or information on animal welfare, there's something out there for everyone.

Documentaries on veganism that you might be interested in:

1. Cowspiracy - The Sustainability Secret - This documentary examines the environmental impact of animal agriculture and the benefits of a plant-based lifestyle.

2. Forks Over Knives - This documentary explores the health benefits of a plant-based diet and examines the science behind it.

3. What the Health - A follow-up to Cowspiracy, this documentary examines the connection between diet and disease.

4. Eating Animals - Based on the book by Jonathan Safran Foer, this documentary explores the ethical and environmental implications of animal agriculture.

5. The Game Changers - This documentary explores the benefits of plant-based eating for athletes and includes interviews with several world-class athletes.

6. Earthlings - This documentary exposes the cruelty of animal farming and the exploitation of animals for food, clothing, and other purposes.

7. Vegan: Everyday Stories - This documentary profiles several individuals who have adopted a vegan lifestyle and explores their motivations and experiences.

8. Vegucated - This documentary follows three meat-loving New Yorkers as they adopt a vegan lifestyle for six weeks.

9. Dominion - This documentary exposes the reality of animal agriculture and features footage from hidden cameras inside slaughterhouses and farms.

10. The Invisible Vegan - This documentary explores the history and cultural significance of veganism within the African American community.

Vegan books out there to read!

Here are just a few recommendations:

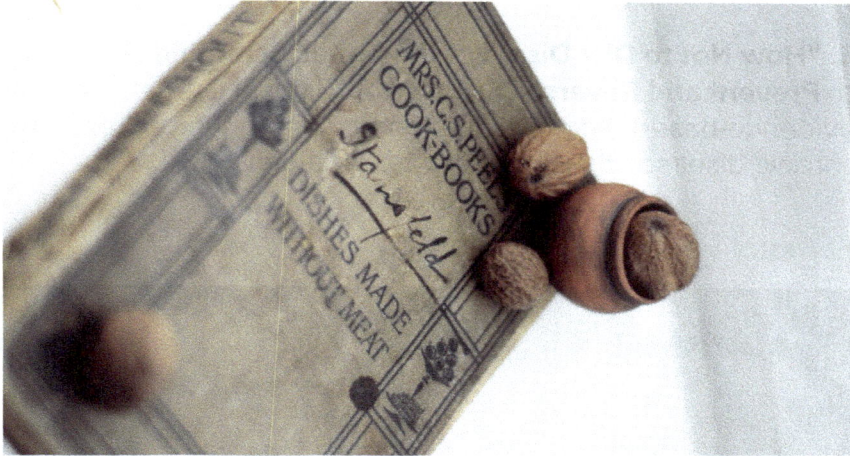

1. "Eating Animals" by Jonathan Safran Foer - This non-fiction book explores the ethical, environmental, and health implications of eating meat.

2. "The China Study" by T. Colin Campbell - This book is based on one of the largest nutrition studies ever conducted and presents compelling evidence for a plant-based diet.

4. "Animal Liberation" by Peter Singer - This classic book is a landmark in the animal rights movement and argues for the moral consideration of animals.

5. "Why We Love Dogs, Eat Pigs, and Wear Cows" by Melanie Joy - This non-fiction book explores the psychological and social reasons why we have different attitudes toward different animals and argues for a vegan lifestyle.

6. "The Omnivore's Dilemma: A Natural History of Four Meals" by Michael Pollan. Explores the food industry and the origins of what we eat.

7. "In Defense of Food: An Eater's Manifesto" by Michael Pollan. Is a book that explores the modern food industry and how it has contributed to the rise of chronic diseases such as obesity, diabetes, and heart disease.

8. "How Not to Die: Discover the Foods Scientifically Proven to Prevent and Reverse Disease" by Michael Greger. Provides evidence-based recommendations for preventing or reversing chronic diseases through a plant-based diet.

Famous Vegans

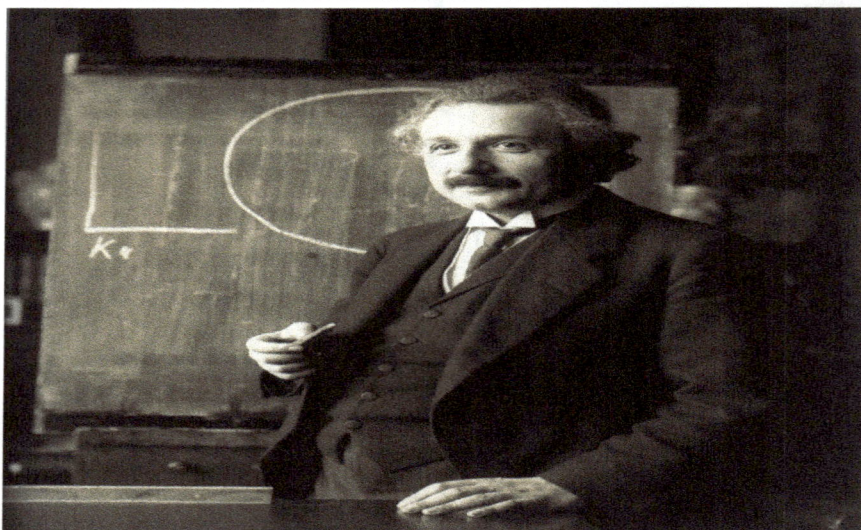

Veganism has become increasingly popular in recent years due to its health benefits and positive impact on the environment. More and more people are recognizing the importance of sustainable living and reducing their carbon footprint, which is why veganism has gained such a strong following in the music industry, professional sports arena and beyond.

Here are just a few:

Some notable examples include Mobb Deep's Prodigy, Wu-Tang Clan's RZA, and Jay-Z. In addition, many other musicians and celebrities have adopted a plant-based lifestyle, including Beyonce, Ariana Grande, and Ellie Goulding.

Albert Einstein - the famous physicist was a lifelong vegetarian and reportedly considered going vegan later in life.

Venus Williams - the professional tennis player adopted a raw vegan diet in 2011 after being diagnosed with an autoimmune disease.

Moby - the musician and DJ has been a vegan for over 30 years and is a passionate animal rights activist.

Joaquin Phoenix - the Oscar-winning actor and animal rights activist has been a vegan since he was three years old.

Bryan Adams - the singer-songwriter has been vegan for over 30 years and is a vocal advocate for animal rights.

Natalie Portman - the actress has been vegan since 2009 and has spoken out about the environmental and health benefits of plant-based eating.

Woody Harrelson - the veteran actor has been vegan for over 30 years and is a well-known environmental activist.

Kyrie Irving - the Brooklyn Nets point guard has been known to follow a vegan diet, incorporating plenty of fruits and vegetables into his meals.

Chris Paul - the Phoenix Suns point guard has also been vocal about his vegan diet, which he says helps him stay in top physical condition.

Damian Lillard - the Portland Trail Blazers point guard is another NBA player who has embraced a plant-based diet, citing health and performance benefits.

JaVale McGee - the Cleveland Cavaliers center has been vegan for several years now and credits the diet with helping him recover from injuries and stay in shape during the off-season.

Wilson Chandler - the Brooklyn Nets forward has also been vegan for a while and has spoken out about the benefits of plant-based eating for both his health and the environment.

Colin Kaepernick - the former NFL quarterback has been vocal about his vegan diet, citing health and ethical reasons for the switch.

LaTocha Scott-Bivens - an American Singer/songwriter and a member of the American R&B group Xscape. Author of a vegan cookbook, "LaTocha's Planted Lifestyle".

Lizzo - an American singer, rapper, and flutist who has gained widespread popularity for her empowering and body-positive music. Is a vegan and has been open about her plant-based lifestyle on social media. She often shares vegan recipes and promotes a healthy and compassionate diet.

Jermaine Dupri - an American rapper, songwriter, and record producer. Owner of vegan Ice-Cream brand "JD's Vegan".

Jessica Chastain -an American actress and producer.

Styles P - an American rapper, author, and entrepreneur. He is a member of the hip hop group The LOX and has released numerous solo albums throughout his career. Styles P is also known for his activism around health and wellness, particularly in the areas of plant-based diets and holistic healing.

RZA - an American rapper, record producer, and actor. He is best known as the founder and leader of the Wu-Tang Clan, a highly influential hip hop group from New York City.

Stevie Wonder - an American singer, songwriter, musician, and record producer. He is considered one of the most influential musicians of the 20th century,

SOURCES

These sources are considered credible because they are reputable organizations with expertise in the field of genetics, agriculture, and food safety.

The World Health Organization (WHO) - https://www.who.int/foodsafety/areas_work/food-technology/faq-genetically-modified-food/en/

The National Academies of Sciences, Engineering, and Medicine - https://www.nap.edu/catalog/23395/genetically-engineered-crops-experiences-and-prospects

The American Association for the Advancement of Science (AAAS) - https://www.aaas.org/topics/genetic-engineering

The Non-GMO Project - https://www.nongmoproject.org/

The Organic Trade Association (OTA) - https://ota.com/food-safety-and-advocacy/organic-fiber-and-food-facts/gmos-and-the-environment

The Center for Food Safety - https://www.centerforfoodsafety.org/issues/311/genetically-engineered-crops/about-genetically-engineered-foods/cross-pollination-contamination

(Source: https://www.heart.org/en/healthy-living/healthy-eating/eat-smart/nutrition-basics/soy-protein)